Practice Pearls in
NEUROLOGY

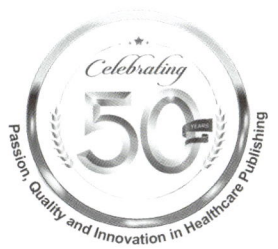

Practice Pearls in NEUROLOGY

Series II

Editors

Bhanu Kesavamurthy MBBS DNB DM FMMC FRCP
Director
Director of Neurology
Dr Mehta's Hospital
Chennai, Tamil Nadu, India

D Vasudevan MD DM
Professor and Head
Department of Neurology
Saveetha Medical College
Chennai, Tamil Nadu, India

AV Srinivasan MD DM PhD FAAN FIAN DSC FRCP
Head of the Department
Institute of Neurology
Madras Medical College and Research Institute
Chennai, Tamil Nadu, India

Foreword
CU Velmurugendran

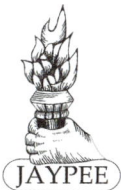

JAYPEE
JAYPEE BROTHERS MEDICAL PUBLISHERS
The Health Sciences Publisher
New Delhi | London | Panama

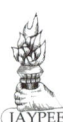

Jaypee Brothers Medical Publishers (P) Ltd

Headquarters
Jaypee Brothers Medical Publishers (P) Ltd
4838/24, Ansari Road, Daryaganj
New Delhi 110 002, India
Phone: +91-11-43574357
Fax: +91-11-43574314
Email: jaypee@jaypeebrothers.com

Overseas Offices

J.P. Medical Ltd
83 Victoria Street, London
SW1H 0HW (UK)
Phone: +44 20 3170 8910
Fax: +44 (0)20 3008 6180
Email: info@jpmedpub.com

Jaypee-Highlights Medical Publishers Inc
City of Knowledge, Bld. 235, 2nd Floor, Clayton
Panama City, Panama
Phone: +1 507-301-0496
Fax: +1 507-301-0499
Email: cservice@jphmedical.com

Jaypee Brothers Medical Publishers (P) Ltd
17/1-B Babar Road, Block-B, Shaymali
Mohammadpur, Dhaka-1207
Bangladesh
Mobile: +08801912003485
Email: jaypeedhaka@gmail.com

Jaypee Brothers Medical Publishers (P) Ltd
Bhotahity, Kathmandu, Nepal
Phone: +977-9741283608
Email: kathmandu@jaypeebrothers.com

Website: www.jaypeebrothers.com
Website: www.jaypeedigital.com

© 2019, Jaypee Brothers Medical Publishers

The views and opinions expressed in this book are solely those of the original contributor(s)/author(s) and do not necessarily represent those of editor(s) of the book.

All rights reserved. No part of this publication may be reproduced, stored or transmitted in any form or by any means, electronic, mechanical, photocopying, recording or otherwise, without the prior permission in writing of the publishers.

All brand names and product names used in this book are trade names, service marks, trademarks or registered trademarks of their respective owners. The publisher is not associated with any product or vendor mentioned in this book.

Medical knowledge and practice change constantly. This book is designed to provide accurate, authoritative information about the subject matter in question. However, readers are advised to check the most current information available on procedures included and check information from the manufacturer of each product to be administered, to verify the recommended dose, formula, method and duration of administration, adverse effects and contraindications. It is the responsibility of the practitioner to take all appropriate safety precautions. Neither the publisher nor the author(s)/editor(s) assume any liability for any injury and/or damage to persons or property arising from or related to use of material in this book.

This book is sold on the understanding that the publisher is not engaged in providing professional medical services. If such advice or services are required, the services of a competent medical professional should be sought.

Every effort has been made where necessary to contact holders of copyright to obtain permission to reproduce copyright material. If any have been inadvertently overlooked, the publisher will be pleased to make the necessary arrangements at the first opportunity. The **CD/DVD-ROM** (if any) provided in the sealed envelope with this book is complimentary and free of cost. **Not meant for sale.**

Inquiries for bulk sales may be solicited at: jaypee@jaypeebrothers.com

Practice Pearls in Neurology—Series II / Bhanu Kesavamurthy, D Vasudevan, AV Srinivasan

First Edition: **2019**

ISBN: 978-93-5270-558-0

Printed at: Samrat Offset Pvt. Ltd.

Dedicated to

Our parents who made us good human beings.
Our teachers who have guided us to become excellent neurophysicians.
Our students and patients who made everything worthwhile.

CONTRIBUTORS

EDITORS

Bhanu Kesavamurthy MBBS DNB DM FMMC FRCP
Director
Director of Neurology
Dr Mehta's Hospital
Chennai, Tamil Nadu, India

D Vasudevan MD DM
Professor and Head
Department of Neurology
Saveetha Medical College
Chennai, Tamil Nadu, India

AV Srinivasan MD DM PhD FAAN FIAN DSC FRCP
Head of the Department
Institute of Neurology
Madras Medical College and Research Institute
Chennai, Tamil Nadu, India

CONTRIBUTING AUTHORS

Pratik Bhattacharya MD MPH
Department of Neurology
St Joseph Mercy Oakland Hospital
Pontiac, Michigan, USA

Jithin A Bose MD
Senior Resident
Department of Neurology
Goverment Medical College
Thanjavur, Tamil Nadu, India

Sarala Govindarajan MD DM
Professor
Department of Neurology
Institute of Neurology
Chennai, Tamil Nadu, India

Harish Jayakumar MD MRCP
Resident
Department of Neurology
Institute of Neurology
Madras Medical College
Chennai, Tamil Nadu, India

Goutam KA MBBS FCPS
Consultant Internist, Bangladesh

Shunmuga S Kanthimathinathan MD DM
Assistant Professor
Department of Neurology
Institute of Neurology
Madras Medical College and
Government General Hospital
Chennai, Tamil Nadu, India

Adhiti Krishnamoorthy MD
Consultant
Department of Internal Medicine
Dr. Mehta's Multispecialty Hospital
Chennai, Tamil Nadu, India

Ramesh Madhavan MD DM FAAN
Director
Department of Neurology
St. Joseph Mercy Oakland Hospital
Pontiac, Michigan, USA

Philo H Philomin MD DM
Assistant Professor
Department of Neurology
Sri Ramachandra Medical College
and Research Institute
Chennai, Tamil Nadu, India

Athi Ponnusamy
MD DM MRCP CCT FRCP (Lond)
FRCP (Glasg)
Consultant Clinical
Neurophysiologist
Department of Clinical
Neurophysiology
Greater Manchester Neuroscience
Centre
Salford Royal NHS Foundation
Trust & Central Manchester
Foundation Trust
Salford, England, United Kingdom

R Raghavendran MBBS MCH
Professor of Neurosuergery
Institute of Neurosurgery
Madras Medical College
Chennai, Tamil Nadu, India

V Rajalakshmi MD
Professor,
Department of Pathology
Esi Medical College and Hospital
Chennai, Tamil Nadu, India

R Lakshminarasimhan
Ranganathan MD DNB DM DNB
Professor
Department of Neurology
Madras Medical College
Chennai, Tamil Nadu, India

Ken Richter DO
Department of Rehabilitation
Medicine
St Joseph Mercy Oakland
Hospital
Pontiac, Michigan, USA

Vinoth K Selvaraj MD DM
Associate Professor
Department of Neurology
Saveetha Medical College
Hospital
Chennai, Tamil, India

J Senthilnathan MD DM
Assistant Professor
Department of Neurology
Sree Balaji Medical College and
Hospital
Chennai, Tamil Nadu, India

Paranjothi Shanmugam
MD DM
Senior Consultant Neurologist and
Former Head
Department of Neurology
Indira Gandhi Government
General Hospital and Post
Graduate Institute
Puducherry, India

M Thangaraj MD DM
Professor and Head
Department of Neurology
Government Thanjavur Medical
College
Thanjavur, Tamil Nadu, India

Suresh C Thirunavukarasu
MD DM
Consultant Neurologist and Head
Department Of Neurology
Indira Gandhi Government
General Hospital and Post
Graduate Institute
Puducherry, India

Meenakshisundaram U MD DM
Senior Consultant and Coordinator
in Neurology, Apollo Hospitals
Chennai, Tamil Nadu, India

Sreenivas UM MD
Resident in Neurology
Madras Medical College
Chennai, Tamil Nadu, India

Poorna J Visa
Clinical Assistant
AVS Clinic
Chennai

FOREWORD

This is a real pearl consisting of many important practical problems, clinical approach thereto, and treatment. Management of neurogenic bladder and carpal tunnel syndrome are of day to day importance. The chapter on bidirectional interaction between sleep and epilepsy is interesting. A long discussed topic on granulomas of the brain is again dealt with in detail.

Management of normal pressure hydrocephalus, nonmotor rehabilitation in stroke, sleep disorders in Parkinson disease, and approach to low backache are essential topics from the practice standpoint. The management of Parkinson disease is highlighted.

The neurological manifestation of thyroid disease is dealt with in detail. The role and relevance of statins in stroke is of current importance. Overall, the contents of this series is of utmost value for the practicing neurologists as well as students and I am sure will be very deeply appreciated by all

CU Velmurugendran
MD DM (Neuro) FAMS FRCP DSc (Hon.Causa)

PREFACE TO SERIES II

The encouraging and enthusiastic reception accorded to Series I of *Practice Pearls in Neurology* by seasoned neurologists and students alike has been the impetus to compile this volume. The principle of addressing topics seldom dealt with in detail in mainstream textbooks, yet of immense importance in day-to-day practice has continued to guide us in this series as well.

The presentations though eclectic, are crisp, practically relevant, and to the point. Needless to say, the vast experience of the faculty has contributed in no small measure to the final product. We hope that Series II will prove as useful as its predecessor in being an immediate source of clinical information and reference for the practicing neurologist. We are grateful to Mr MB Kumaresh Menon and Ms Barkha Arora at Jaypee Brothers Medical Publishers (P) Ltd. for their perseverance and help in ensuring that this Series is readied in time for publication. We are thankful to our families for their encouragement and support throughout.

Bhanu Kesavamurthy
D Vasudevan
AV Srinivasan

PREFACE TO SERIES I

Practice Pearls in Neurology has been conceived and executed as a unique compilation of the topics elaborated in the annual seminars which go by the same name. These seminars have been conducted over the past three years and will be continued in the years to come. The abiding principle of these day long seminars have been to present commonly encountered (but seldom dealt with in standard books in a practically useful manner) conditions, in such a way as to help the novice as well as the adept. The presentations are aimed at focusing on knowledge or experience crystallized over the years into valuable pearls of wisdom pertaining to the topics under consideration.

A galaxy of teachers with rich clinical experience are the faculty for these seminars. This compilation of select topics gleaned from the collection forms Series 1 of the Practice Pearls in Neurology Series. The contributing authors have dealt with their respective topics in a succinct and exemplary manner. We are grateful to all the authors for both their excellent contribution and their patience. We are especially delighted that the doyen of neurology, Professor CU Velmurugendran agreed to write the foreword for this book. We are grateful to Mr MB Kumaresh menon and Ms Sheetal Arora at Jaypee Brothers Medical Publishers for their help. We are thankful to our families for their constant support.

AV Srinivasan
D Vasudevan
K Bhanu

CONTENTS

1. Management of Neurogenic Bladder 1
   M Thangaraj, Jithin A Bose

2. Clinical Approach to Carpal Tunnel Syndrome 12
   Bhanu Kesavamurthy, Senthil Nathan

3. Bidirectional Interaction Between Sleep and Epilepsy: Practice Points 22
   Athi Ponnusamy

4. Granulomas of Nontuberculous and Noncystisercal Origin 32
   Suresh C Thirunavukarasu, Paranjothi Shanmugam

5. Management of Normal Pressure Hydrocephalus 57
   Sarala Govindarajan, Harish Jayakumar, Shunmuga S Kanthimathinathan,
   R Lakshminarasimhan Ranganathan

6. Nonmotor Rehabilitation in Stroke 65
   Philo H Philomin, Bhanu Kesavamurthy

7. Sleep Disorders in Parkinson's Disease: From Research to Clinical Practice 73
   Vinoth K Selvaraj

8. Approach to Evaluation and Management of Low Back Ache 79
   R Raghavendran

9. Management of Parkinson Disease in This Millennium 91
   Goutam KA, AV Srinivasan, Poorna J Visa, V Rajalakshmi

10. Neurological Manifestations of Thyroid Disorders 107
    Adhiti Krishnamoorthy

11. Stroke and Motor Recovery 116
    Ken Richter, Pratik Bhattacharya, Ramesh Madhavan

12. Current Role of Statins in Cerebrovascular Diseases 123
    Meenakshisundaram U, Sreenivas UM

    Index 129

PLATE 1

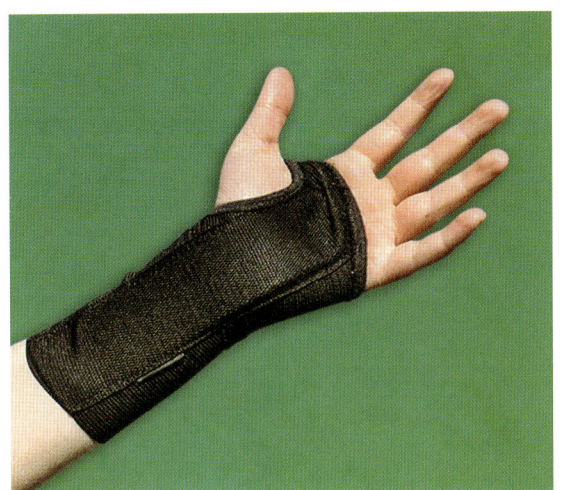

FIG. 4: Splinting. *(Chapter 2)*

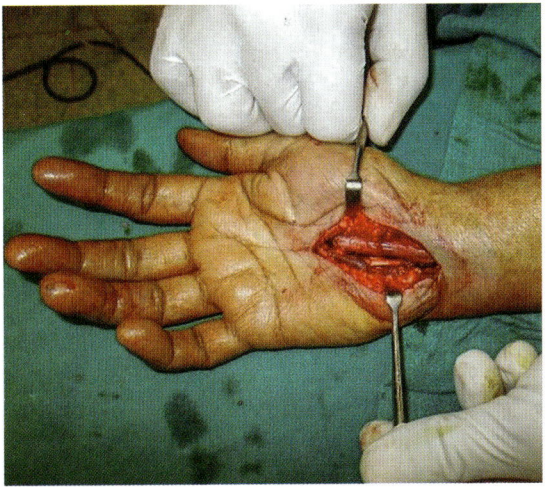

FIG. 5: Surgical decompression of carpal tunnel. *(Chapter 2)*

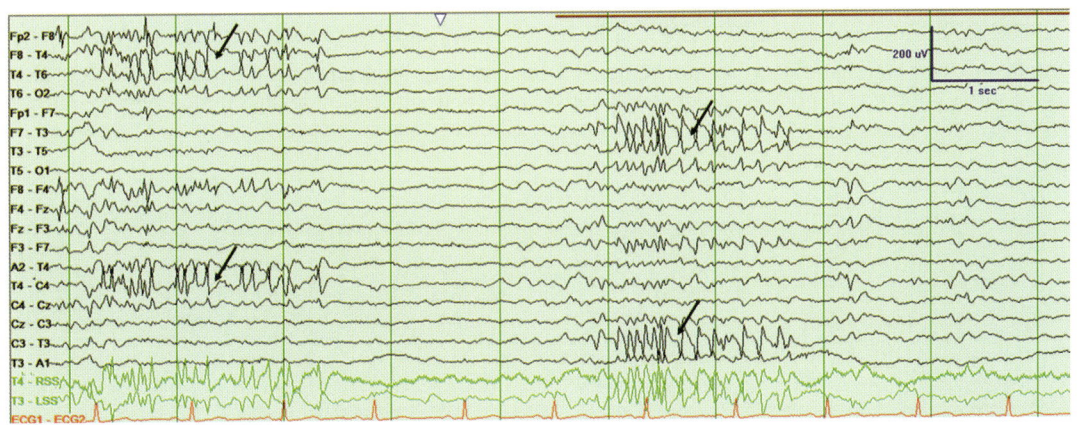

FIG. 1: Potentiation of spike wave discharges over temporal regions independently in slow wave sleep in a case of bitemporal temporal lobe epilepsy. *(Chapter 3)*

PLATE 2

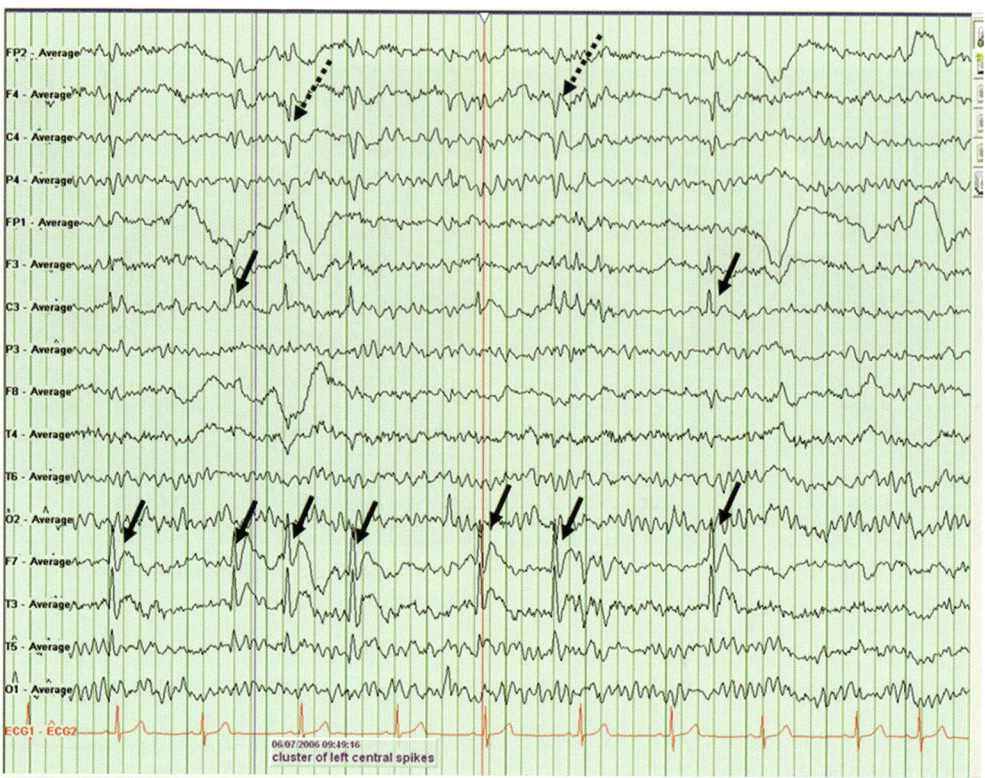

FIG. 2: Centro temporal spikes in a child with benign Rolandic epilepsy: Black arrows and dotted arrows highlight the negative spikes in centro temporal electrodes and positive spikes in frontal electrodes in common average derivation. *(Chapter 3)*

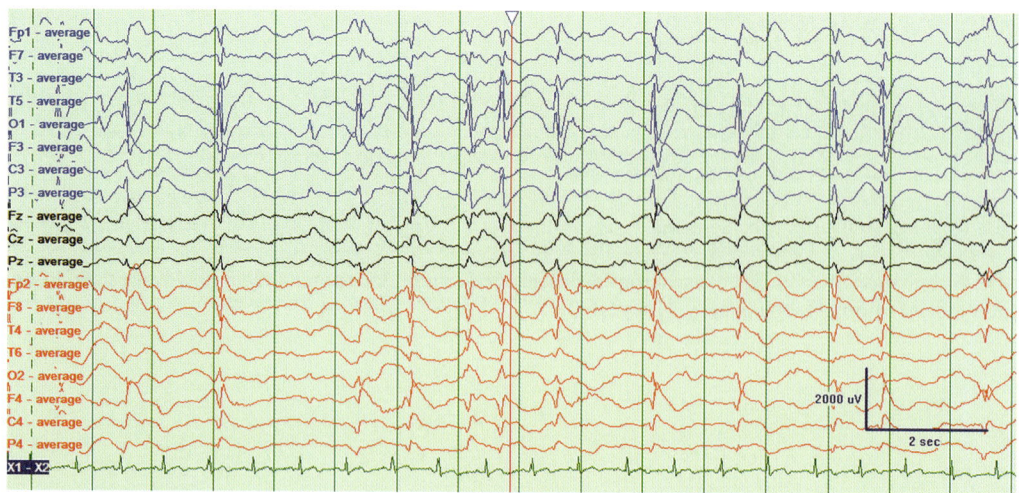

FIG. 3: Electrical status in slow wave sleep. If clinical features support global cognitive decline, diagnosis of continuous spike in slow wave sleep is diagnosed. *(Chapter 3)*

PLATE 3

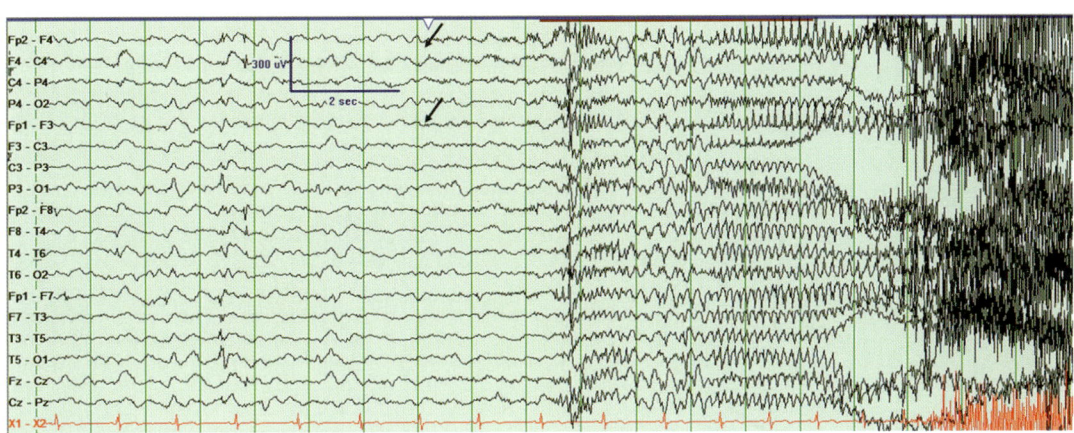

FIG. 4: Ictal scalp electroencephalography in a patient with genetic generalized epilepsy during one generalized tonic clonic seizure from slow-wave sleep. Black arrow corresponds to ictal onset with subsequent classic ictal evolution. *(Chapter 3)*

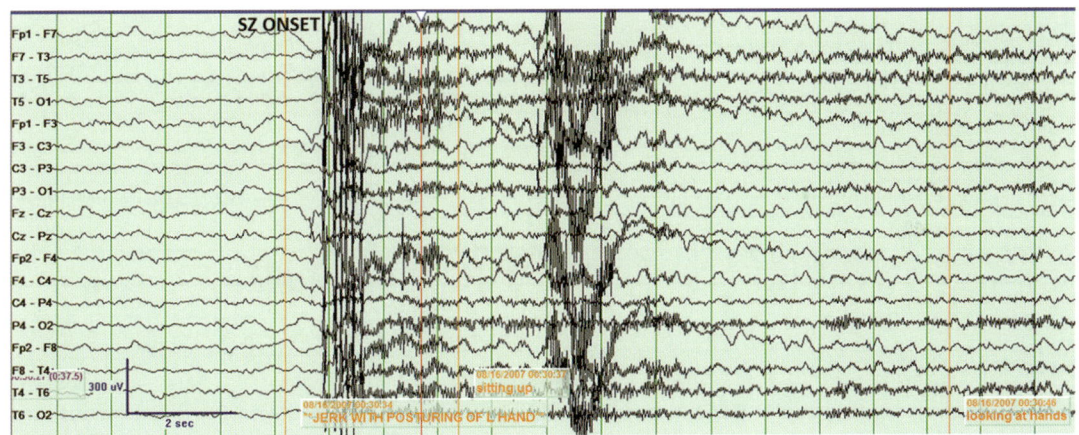

FIG. 5: Ictal scalp electroencephalography in a patient with nocturnal frontal lobe seizure during one brief clonic with asymmetric tonic seizure from slow-wave sleep. Note nonlocalized and nonlateralized ictal scalp electroencephalography pattern. (Semiology in video may be useful for localization and lateralization). *(Chapter 3)*

PLATE 4

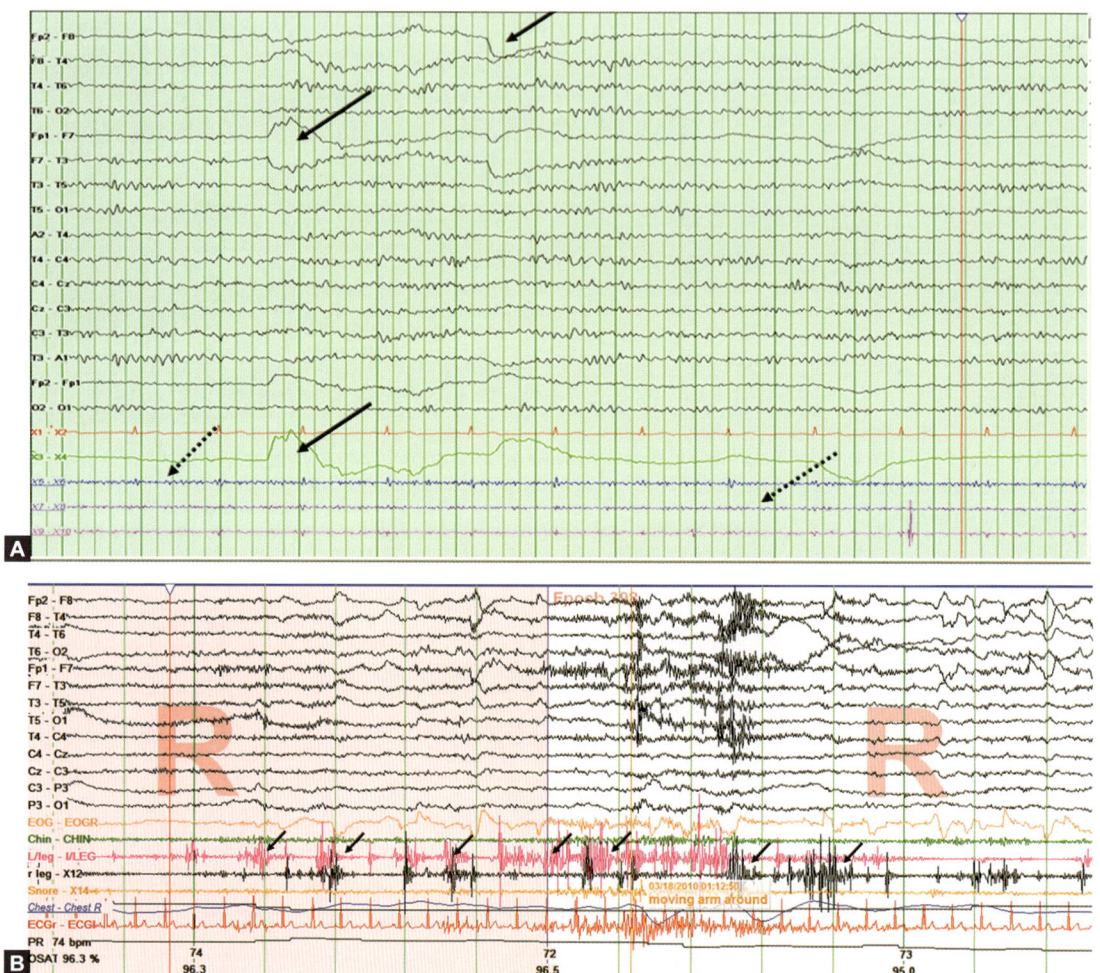

FIG. 6: **A,** Electroencephalography (EEG) in normal rapid eye movement (REM) sleep. Black continuous arrows show some of the rapid eye movements in electrooculography and EEG; black dotted arrows highlight loss of electromyography (EMG) tone; **B,** EEG during REM behavior disorder. Black arrows show lack of atonia in EMG and increased EMG activity due to dream enacting behavior. EEG shows desynchronized normal pattern with no ictal epileptic rhythm. *(Chapter 3)*

PLATE 5

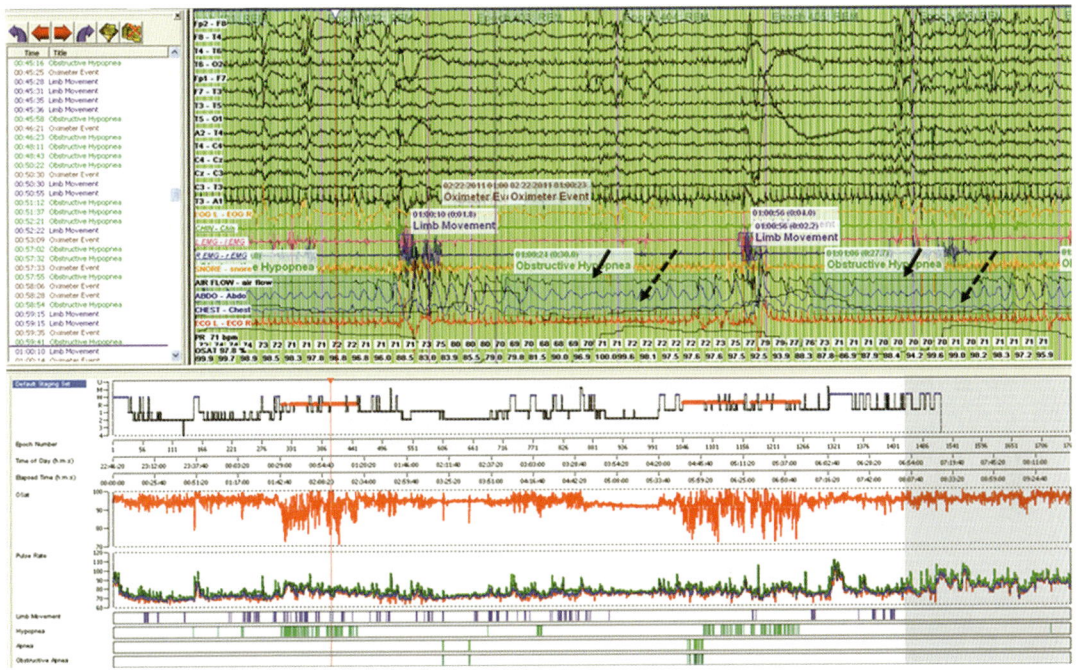

FIG. 7: An example slide for overnight polysomnography with hypnogram. Black arrows show absence of nasal airflow and dotted arrows show continuing chest and abdominal movements. This is typical pattern for obstructive sleep apnea. In central apnea, both airflow and chest/abdominal movements will be flat and unreactive during the periods of apnea. *(Chapter 3)*

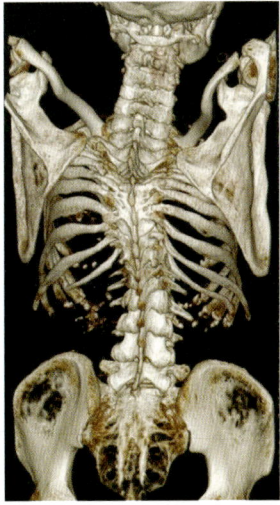

FIG 14: 3D reconstructed computed tomography image exquisitely demonstrating kyphoscoliosis. *(Chapter 8)*

CHAPTER 1

Management of Neurogenic Bladder

M Thangaraj, Jithin A Bose

INTRODUCTION

Neurogenic bladder (NB) or neurogenic lower urinary tract dysfunction (NLUTD), a dysfunction of the urinary bladder and urethra due to disease of the central or peripheral nervous system. Various neurological diseases like stroke, dementias, Parkinson's disease, spinal injuries, spinal tumors, congenital lesions like spinal dysraphism and diabetes can produce NB/NLUTD. The neurogenic dysfunction manifest as over active or underactive bladder which depends on extent and level of neural lesion. It is not only a medical problem but also a major social issue.[1]

ANATOMY OF BLADDER INNERVATION (FIG. 1)

Autonomic Innervation:
- Parasympathetic: S2- S4 motor to detrusor, inhibitory to internal sphincter
- Sympathetic: D10-L2 motor to sphincter, inhibitory to detrusor
- Origin: Intermediolateral grey column.

Somatic:
- Pudendal nerve (S2, S3, S4)
- Origin: Nucleus of Onuf/Ventral horn.

Cortical Micturition Center:
- Second frontal gyrus (Paracentral lobule) inhibitory to PMC.

Pontine Micturition Centre:
- Supraspinal regulation of micturition.

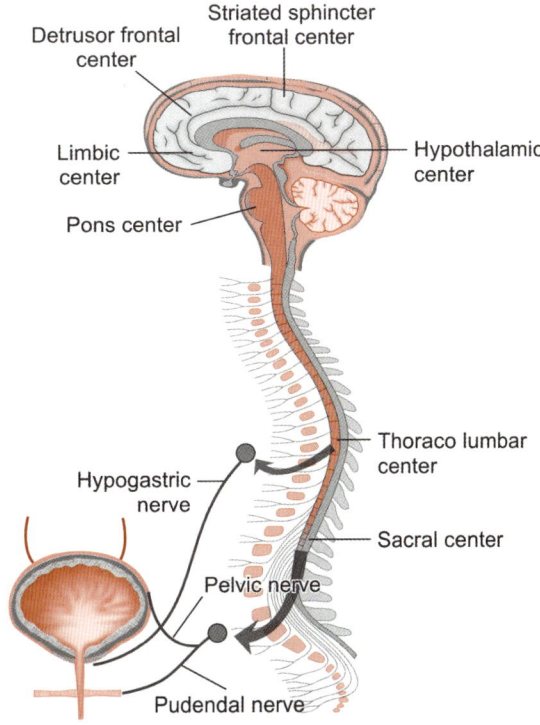

FIG. 1: Anatomy of bladder innervation.

Briefly, neurologic voiding dysfunctions can be classified as (Fig. 2):
- Suprapontine lesions
- Suprasacral spinal cord lesions
- Sacral spinal cord lesions
- Cauda equina and pelvic plexus lesions.

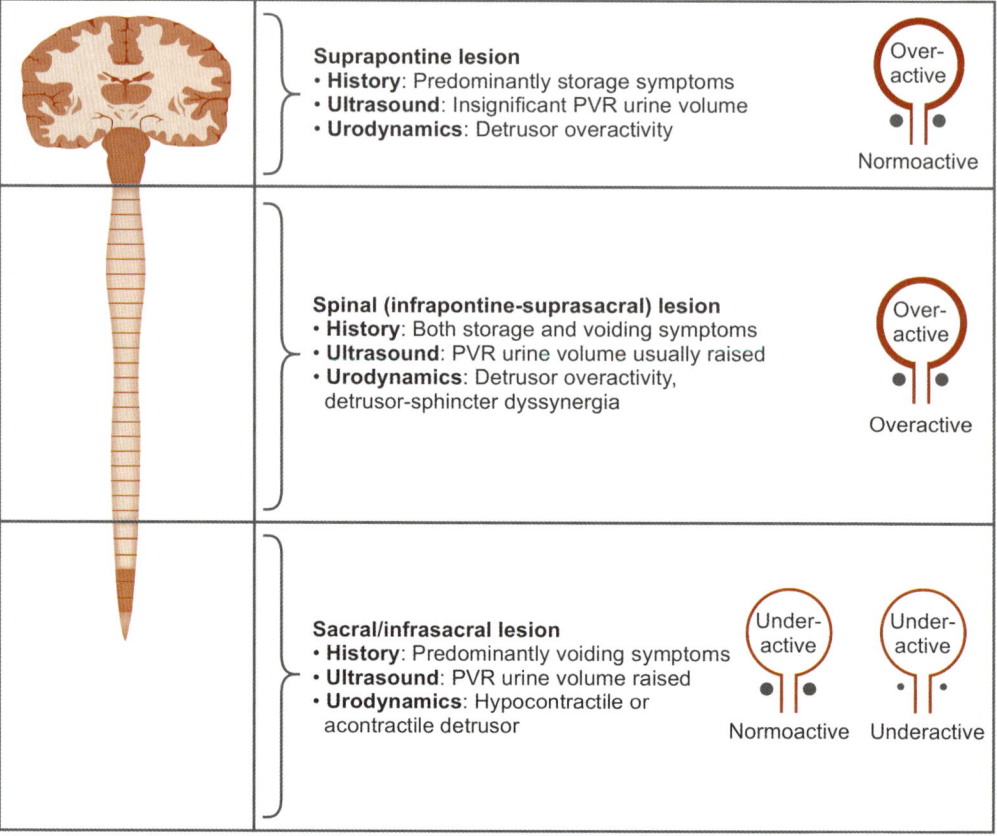

PVR, postvoid residual.
FIG. 2: Bladder dysfunction due to lesions at various levels.

The suprapontine areas are responsible for providing inhibitory signals to the pontine micturition center, which provides signals for regulating micturition. Suprapontine lesions such as dementias, CVAs, and brain tumors can therefore cause loss in inhibitory signals to the pontine center, resulting in urinary frequency, urgency, urge incontinence, and uninhibited voiding. But there is no impact on the coordination of the bladder and sphincter.

Suprasacral spinal cord lesions result in the loss of supraspinal input. This loss of input typically results in uncontrolled activation of the micturition reflex, via afferent fiber stimulation, causing uninhibited detrusor contractions. Signals from the pons that help to coordinate bladder and sphincter activity can be affected, resulting in detrusor-sphincter dyssynergia (DSD). Detrusor-sphincter dyssynergia occurs more frequently with higher spinal lesions.

Sacral spinal cord lesions can manifest with varying degrees of upper and lower motor neuron damage. This can result in different clinical manifestations, including detrusor hyper-reflexia and areflexia. Similarly, the external sphincter can be affected in different ways, ranging from complete loss of function to DSD.

Lesions that are distal to the sacral spinal cord, such as those present in myelodysplasia, cauda equina injury, radical pelvic surgery, or pelvic plexus injury can result in an areflexic, hypotonic, or flaccid bladder and a denervated sphincter. The external sphincter can be in a fixed position, resulting in chronic obstruction and consequent loss of bladder compliance.

Functional Classification of Neurogenic Bladder Dysfunction (Box 1)

The functional system is perhaps the most simple and widely accepted classification system for lower urinary tract disorders. First proposed by F. Brantley Scott's group in 1968,[2] this system was later popularized by Alan J. Wein.[3] In its essence, this system describes whether the deficit is primarily one of:
- The filling/storage or
- The emptying/voiding phases of micturition.

A failure of filling/storage and failure of emptying/voiding can result from either bladder or outlet abnormalities, or a combination of both.

Lapides Classification of Neurogenic Bladder[4] (Table 1)

This classification is useful and easy for understanding and remembering. But some patient may not fit into any one category.

EVALUATION (TABLE 2)

As always the patient history is an essential part of the diagnosis. Duration and level of lesion and previous medical histories are important data. The special history includes a complete review on the general neurological, specific somatic and sensory, urinary, anorectal, sexual, gynecological symptoms and signs. Sensations of bladder filling have to be asked for. Autonomic dysreflexia has to be investigated if a spinal lesion above T6 has occurred. The way bladder emptying has been done so far, the eventual presence of incontinence, and any usage of catheter or

Box 1: Functional classification in neurologic disorders

Failure to store
- Because of the bladder
  - Detrusor hyper-reflexia (neurogenic detrusor overactivity)
  - Impaired contractility
- Because of the outlet
  - Neurogenic intrinsic sphincter deficiency

Failure to empty
- Because of the bladder
  - Impaired contractility
  - Detrusor areflexia
- Because of the outlet
  - Detrusor-external sphincter dyssynergia
  - Bladder neck dyssynergia

Table 1: Lapides classification of neurogenic bladder

Type	Pathogenesis	Possible etiology	Symptoms
Sensory	Damage to sensory fibers from bladder to spinal cord	Diabetes mellitus, pernicious anemia, advanced syphilis	No bladder sensation. Eventual loss of motor function
Motor	Damage to motor fibers from spinal cord to bladder	Herpes zoster, pelvic trauma, surgery	Normal sensation. Failure of motor function
Autonomous	Damage to both motor and spinal fibers between bladder and spinal cord	Pelvic trauma, low myelomeningocele, surgery	Failure to generate bladder contraction, loss of bladder sensation
Uninhibited	Injury to cortical regulation of bladder reflex	Stroke, brain tumor cortical trauma	Normal sensation and motor function urge incontinence, urinary frequency
Reflex	Damage to spinal cord between sacrum and brainstem	Spinal cord injury, myelomeningocele, transverse myelitis	Poorly coordinated bladder function, loss of sensation, incontinence

Table 2: Important investigations in patients with neurogenic bladder	
Tests	Uses
Urinalysis with cytology and culture	• Helps to find urinary tract infection, • Hematuria, urinary casts etc. and will help in planning additional investigations like cystoscopy
Renal function studies	Blood urea nitrogen and creatinine helps to assess renal function and renal failure
Voiding diary	Records the patient's bladder activity. It gives information about voiding pattern, incontinent episodes, and provocative events
The pad test	Objective test that documents and quantifies urine loss and the severity of incontinence
Postvoid residual bladder volume (PVR)	PVR tells about under active detrusor or outlet obstruction. Both of these conditions produces urinary retention with overflow incontinence
Uroflow rate	• Uroflow is a simple non-invasive urodynamic measurement. It measures the volume/time of urine accumulation. Combined with PVR, it is an excellent screening test for bladder outlet obstruction and LUTS (Lower Urinary tract symptoms) • Low uroflow rate indicates urethral obstruction, weak detrusor, or combination of both
Filling cystometrogram (CMG)	Provides information on bladder storage capacity, sensation, compliance of bladder (ability to expand during increasing volume of urine), presence or absence of detrusor over activity
Voiding CMG	Records the voiding detrusor pressure and the rate of urinary flow. Only test available to assess bladder contractility and the severity of a bladder outlet obstruction can be combined with video urodynamic study and voiding cystogram in complicated cases of incontinence
Static cystogram	Helps to confirm the presence of stress incontinence, the degree of urethral motion, cystocele and vesico-vaginal fistula or bladder diverticulum
Electromyography (EMG)	EMG allows accurate diagnosis of the detrusor sphincter dyssynergia that is common in spinal cord injuries
Cystoscopy	• Allows discovery of bladder lesions (e.g., bladder cancer, bladder stone) that would remain undiagnosed by urodynamics alone. • Indicated in persistent irritative voiding symptoms or hematuria
Video urodynamics	• Video urodynamics is the criterion standard for evaluation of a patient with incontinence. Video urodynamics combines the radiographic findings of voiding cystourethrogram and multichannel urodynamics • Video urodynamics enables documentation of lower urinary tract anatomy, such as vesicoureteral reflux and bladder diverticulum, as well as the functional pressure-flow relationship between the bladder and the urethra

appliances are important. Evaluation following soinal cord injury is summarized in flow chart 1.

MANAGEMENT

The main objectives for current strategies in the management of NB are:

- Protection of the upper urinary tract
- Restoration of the lower urinary tract function
- Improvement of urinary continence
- Improvement of the patient's quality of life (QoL).

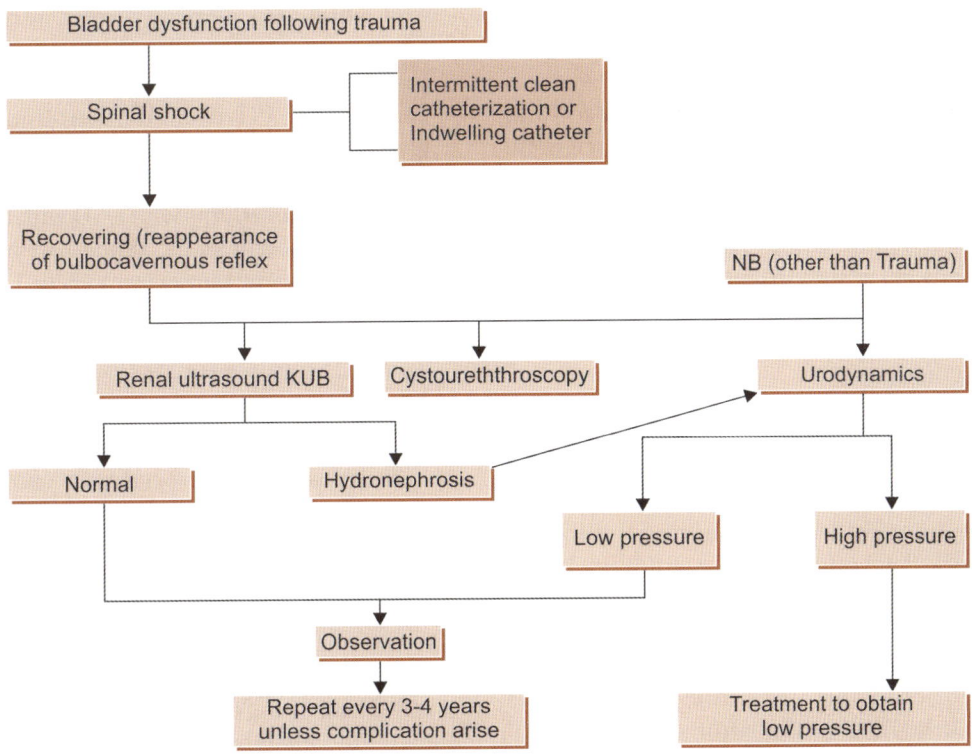

NB, neurogenic bladder; KUB, kidney ureters bladder.
FLOWCHART 1: Diagnosis and follow-up of patients with neurogenic bladder dysfunction.

Conservative Treatment

Most widely applied treatment modality in NB. Conservative treatment is cheap, easily available even in periphery where urologists not available with less complications. The goals are to achieve a good bladder storage/voiding cycle, with low intravesical pressure with maintenance of urinary continence and little or no residual urine. These techniques includes:
- Behavioral techniques
- Physiotherapy
- Intermittent catheterization and intermittent self-catheterization
- Transurethral and suprapubic catheters
- Appliances (condom catheters and penile clamp).

Behavioral Techniques

Behavioral therapy is important in all patients. It is most valuable in patients with some amount of bladder control and intact bladder sensation. It is helpful in patients like CVA, multiple sclerosis (MS), dementia, Parkinson's, incomplete spinal cord injury (SCI) and transverse myelitis.

- *Timed voiding:* Chronic/frequent over distension leads to flaccid, large capacity, permanent paralytic bladder. Timed voiding means maintaining fixed interval between episodes of urination/toileting. The primary goal of timed voiding is to void before urinary urgency and occurrence of incontinence. It is done by frequent voiding to lower the residual urine or by increasing the voiding interval to reduce frequency. This type of "bladder drill" helps to hold more urine and inhibit inappropriate detrusor contractions during the filling phase of bladder
- *Modifying/Adapting drinking habits:* Includes balanced fluid intake/restricting caffeinated beverages and bladder irritants.

Toilet facility should be nearby to the patient which improves the mobility. Planning a fluid schedule is an important initial event in the management. The recommended fluid schedule is 400 cc with meals; 200 cc at 10 AM, 2 PM, and 4 PM; and only sips of fluid after the evening meal (1800 cc/day total). This schedule limits the urine formation about 1500 cc with insensible fluid loss.

Patient is also instructed to keep a voiding diary—helps to know functional bladder capacity, sensation.

Physiotherapy

Detrusor over activity from defective central inhibition or increased detrusor afferent activity can be improved by reinforcing inhibitory pathways. Pelvic floor muscle training should benefit patients with weak pelvic musculature. To activate this myotomes a simple technique like standing on tiptoes can suppress urgency.[5]

The activation of sacral dermatomes particularly glans penis, clitoris and anus can inhibit detrusor activity by enhancing sympathetic neurons and inhibiting preganglionic bladder motor neurons.

The bladder drill for urgency and urge incontinence, consists of teaching the patients to sit down on a rolled-up towel and press on or squeeze the clitoris/glans penis to activate the appropriate dermatomes. This type of training reduces urgency by inhibiting the bladder contraction and increase the functional bladder capacity.

Transcutaneous electrical nerve stimulation over sacral dermatomes (s2-s4) reduces urgency and urge incontinence. Various studies proved that electrode placed over s3 dermatome and stimulation of this electrodes in the range of 2-10 Hz has shown significant positive response in the form of reduction in bladder urgency, improvement in bladder capacity and reduction of bladder pressure compared to pre-stimulation.

- *Physiotherapy for detrusor hypoactivity*: Detrusor overactivity can be enhanced by pressing or tapping over the bladder wall which will activate stretch receptors. Other techniques like bending forward and straining can also activate bladder contraction. Pelvic floor relaxation helps bladder emptying.

Pelvic floor muscle electric stimulation is very useful in patients with DSD with urinary retention. Plevnik et al.[6] treated six patients with spinal cord lesions from C5 to T4, using anal or vaginal electrodes monophasic square pulses of 1 ms, frequency of 20 Hz and 50–90 mA, a reduction in maximal urethral pressure was reported.

Intravesical transurethral bladder stimulation uses the procedure of combining direct stimulation of bladder receptors with visual feedback using patient observance of cystometric pressure changes. It is useful in patients with bladder underactivity due to neuromuscular weakness

- *Triggered reflex voiding*: It consists of bladder reflex triggering maneuvers performed by patient to elicit reflex detrusor contractions by external stimuli. These are suprapubic tapping, thigh scratching, squeezing the glans penis and the scrotal skin, pulling on the crines pubis, anal/rectal manipulation. Only in a minority these methods are useful
- *Bladder expression:* Comprises various maneuvers like Valsalva (abdominal straining) and the Credé (manual compression of the lower abdomen) maneuvers. These methods are useful in patients with lower motor neuron lesions where combination of an underactive detrusor with an underactive sphincter or with an incompetent urethral closure mechanism of other origin.

Catheterization

Intermittent Catheterization and Self Intermittent Catheterization

The aim of catheterization is mainly to evacuate the bladder. In NB with partial or complete urinary retention intermittent catheterization (IC) is the technique of choice. Self-administered IC improves patient self-care, independence, decreases barriers to sexual function and daily activity. For achieving continence in patient on IC a bladder with adequate capacity, low pressure and a balance between fluid intake, residual urine and catheterization frequency is necessary. If the patient retains some voluntary control, voiding can be attempted at timed intervals or when the urge occurs. Intermittent catheterization partly aids in bladder retraining by gradually decreasing residual urine. Complications includes bacteriuria and urinary tract infection (UTI), urethritis, epididymitis, epididymorchitis, prostatitis, urethral trauma, hematuria, urethral false passages, strictures etc. Asymptomatic bacteriuria is a common finding.

In patients whom IC is not feasible, indwelling catheter may be used. This can be urethral catheter or suprapubic catheter. Commonest complication during indwelling catheter are UTIs but in a long term care setting prophylaxis against UTI is usually not advised.

Fluid intake should be generous in patients with indwelling Foleys catheter or suprapubic catheter. Long term catheterization produce bacterial colonization (biofilm) particularly at the catheter tip. Urease producing organisms elevate pH and cause calcium magnesium phosphate crystals leading to catheter obstruction. This produces or aggravates urinary tract infection. To prevent this complications urine pH must be kept alkaline (pH 8), combined with liberal fluid intake (total intake 3L/day). Increasing dietary citrate (fruit juices) to at least 11 g/day helps to keep urine pH 8 in conjunction with increasing fluid intake. Suprapubic catheter has many advantages.
- Easy to maintain catheter and hygiene
- Less tendency to kink
- Less interference with social functioning like sexual activity
- Urethral injury like erosion avoided.

Suprapubic Cystostomy
This technique is mainly used in patients with poor upper extremity dexterity, as well as the presence of DSD. Other potential candidates include patients with extensive urethral damage or in whom other methods are impractical.

Although open suprapubic cystostomy under anesthesia is the definitive gold-standard approach, many less invasive techniques are also available.

Appliances
Condom catheters have a role in male patients with NB for short term management. In the long run, their use may lead to bacteriuria. If applied properly complications are less. In this method frequent change of condom, maintenance of good hygiene, and low bladder pressure is essential. Complications like skin maceration and ulcers may develop but compared with urethral catheters there is low incidence of infections.

PHARMACOLOGIC THERAPIES FOR NEUROGENIC BLADDER (TABLES 3 AND 4)
Many drugs are available for NB, these include:
- Antimuscarinics
- Alpha-blockers
- Tricyclic antidepressants.

Most commonly used are antimuscarinics, mostly administered orally, rarely as intravesical instillation.

Antimuscarinics
Antimuscarinic drugs are the first-line drugs for patients with NB/neurogenic detrusor overactivity (NDO). Acetylcholine is

Table 3: Antimuscarinic drugs

Medication	Dosage
Oxybutynin	2.5– 5mg/day 2–4 times/day
Oxybutynin extended release	5–30 mg once daily (OD)
Tolterodine	1–2 mg two times a day (BD)
Tolterodine extended release	2–4 mg OD
Darifenacin	7.5–15 mg OD
Solifenacin	5–10 mg OD
Trospium chloride	20 mg BD
Trospium chloride extended release	60 mg OD

Table 4: Other drugs used in neurogenic bladder

Drug	Remarks	Therapeutic use	Side effect
Cholinergic agonists: Urecholine	Administered 1 h before bedtime with voiding attempt by manual technique	Promote detrusor contraction in mixed type of NB	Hypotension, bradycardia, bronchospasm abdominal cramps
Alpha 2 adrenergic agonists: Clonidine, tizanidine	Tizanidine oral Clonidine: Oral and transdermal	For reducing bladder outflow resistance and also reduce pain and skeletal muscle tone	Fatigue, dizziness, dry mouth constipation
Alpha 1 adrenergic antagonists: Dibenzyline, terazosin,tTamsulosin, alfuzosin	–	Reduces urinary outflow resistance by post synaptic block	May produce headache, light headedness
Benzodiazepines: Diazepam (potentiate the inhibitory neurotransmitter GABA)	–	To reduce external urinary sphincter spasticity in UMN or mixed lesions	Sedation, delirium, respiratory depression, constipation. Can produce dependence
GABA-B agonists: Baclofen	Modulation of GABA-B receptors at spinal and supraspinal level Can be administered intrathecally	To reduce external urinary sphincter spasticity	Excessive sedation, no dependence compared to diazepam
Vanilloids: Capsaicin/RTX (resiniferatoxin)	Reduces detrusor over activity by desensitizing the unmyelinated c fiber which transmit urothelial pain	Reduces detrusor hyperreflexia in spinal cord lesion	Clinical use is limited because of lack of stability of vanilloid solutions

GABA, gamma-aminobutyric acid; NB, neurogenic bladder; UNM, upper motor neurons.

the neurotransmitter involved in detrusor contractions, antimuscarinics inhibit at muscarinic receptor level leading to relaxation of detrusor and improved storage. This results increased bladder capacity and reduced urgency to void.

Oxybutynin is available as immediate, sustained-release oral preparations, transdermal and topical gels. Tolterodine tartrate and trospium chloride are available both immediate, and sustained-release oral formulation. Since these drugs doesn't cross blood-brain barrier they produce less cognitive side effects and dry mouth than oxybutynin.[7]

Overall, antimuscarinic therapy can provide substantial benefits to patients with NB and NDO. A recent meta-analysis that included a total of 960 patients with NDO in 16 randomized clinical trials (RCTs) found that antimuscarinics were associated with statistically significant better patient-reported cure or improvement, higher maximum cystometric capacity, higher volume at first detrusor contraction and lower maximum detrusor pressure when compared with placebo. Of all these drugs studied and found to be effective no one drug is superior over other. The side effects include dry mouth, constipation, nausea, and visual disturbance.

Combination therapy is considered when monotherapy has failed. Combination of two antimuscarinics at high-dosage was found to be useful when one agent has failed.

Tricyclic Antidepressant Drugs

Introduced for depressive treatment, their side effect made them second line agents. The anticholinergic side-effects of this class of drugs have been used to reduce bladder detrusor tone in neurogenic bladder dysfunction. Imipramine has strong anticholinergic effects, so it reduces bladder tone, increases internal sphincter tone which will facilitate urine storage. Amitriptyline is also used some times.

Botulinum toxin

A naturally occurring neurotoxin, derived from clostridium botulinum bacterium which produce flaccid paralysis of striated muscle by blocking presynaptic release of acetylcholine. Even though many type of botulinum toxin are available commercially, for urological condition onabotulinumtoxinA (BoNT/A) is the FDA-approved one.[8]

The toxin has effect mainly on efferent muscle contraction, with possible afferent effects on bladder function as well.

Injection of BoNT/A into the detrusor muscle produce dose-dependent muscle relaxation due to reduced neural signal transmission. The BoNT/A's effect on bladder smooth muscle is significantly longer than skeletal muscle. Multiple studies confirmed its effect on NB, urinary incontinence, and QoL in MS and SCI patients. At present BoNT/A is approved for patients with detrusor over activity and patients who have poor response to antimuscarinic drugs. The doses used are 200 U to 300 U. Between the used doses both are well tolerated and equally effective. The commonest adverse effect is urinary infections and urinary retention. Increased risk of retention is seen in patients who didn't perform interstitial cystitis at baseline. A dose of 200 U is commonly used because of less adverse effects.[9]

SURGICAL INTERVENTIONS IN NEUROGENIC BLADDER (TABLE 5)

When pharmacological and conservative managements fail surgical options can be considered. It can be of help in many ways like:
- Procedure to enhance detrusor storage
- Procedure to enhance emptying
- Bladder sphincter procedure to restrict emptying
- Bladder sphincter procedure to enhance emptying.

Table 5: Surgical interventions

	Mechanism	Use	Remarks	Complication
Neuromodulation	Enhance detrusor storage by stimulation of Sacral nerve root	Neurogenic Detrusor over activity	Longp-term efficacy is not proved	Lead migration and pain at site of implant
Enterocystoplasty	Enhance detrusor storage by anastomosing ileum or ileocecal segment to detrusor	To increase reservoir and reduce detrusor pressure	Most accepted method for achieving adequate reservoir with success rate of 95%	Infection, anastomotic leaks, enteric or urinary fistulas, strictures
Urinary diversion	Procedure to control detrusor emptying	Patient with NB who have Impractical self-catheterization. Abdominal stoma is created is for clear IC	–	Major Abdominal surgery
Sphincterotomy	Enhance emptying	Reducing urinary outlet obstruction. DSD with hydronephrosis, VUR. Recurrent UTI due to poor bladder emptying. Usually reserved for quadriplegic male	Fewer UTI Incidence, 50% success rate	Haemorrhage during surgery, erectile dysfunction In males, urethral stricture

IC, intermittent catheterization; UTI, urinary tract infection; VUR, vesicoureteral reflux.

Table 6: Future developments

Procedure	Technique	Usefulness
Lumbar to sacral nerve rerouting	Restoring bladder function in spina bifida by creation of a skin-central nervous system bladder reflex arc via lumbar (L5 motor) to sacral (S3) nerve rerouting	• Success rate of 87% in 110 children in China • One-year results of the first North American trial were reported, with 7/9 (87%) of spina bifida
Spinal cord regeneration with fibroblasts transplantation	Transplantation of neuronal and glial precursors into the spinal cord lesions in experimentally induced rats	Reported to result in decreased detrusor pressures and less frequent detrusor hyper reflexia episodes
Implantation of neurotrophin- secreting Schwann cells into rat spinal cord lesions	Implantation of neurotrophin-secreting Schwann cells into rat spinal cord lesions one hour after induced thoracic cord injury	Improved bladder morphology and bladder capacity-Park et al.[10,11]
Olfactory ensheathing cells (OECs)	Glial cells derived from the olfactory placode, have axonal growth promoting properties in their interaction with astrocytes	In a pilot study of 30 human subjects with chronic paraplegia or tetraplegia, Lima et al.[12] transplanted olfactory mucosal cell auto grafts into the area of prior cord damage with at least 1-year (and average of over 2-year) follow up. American Spinal Cord American Spinal Cord Injury Association scores improved in 11 subjects but declined in one, and urodynamic responses were reported improved in five subjects

Some future developments in management is summarized in table 6.

CONCLUSION

Neurological disorders often cause bladder and bowel dysfunction. Most patients with NB need long term or even life-long care for optimal life expectancy and QoL. Timely recognition and treatment are essential to prevent upper and lower urinary tract damage. Evaluation of NB include detailed history, neurological assessment and appropriate investigations including urodynamic study. The neurourological management must be individualized to the patient's needs which often requires multi-disciplinary approach. Before major surgical intervention noninvasive and conservative therapies must be tried. Individual's sexual and fertility function should not be ignored.

REFERENCES

1. Liao L. Evaluation and management of neurogenic bladder: What is new in China? Int J Mol Sci. 2015;16(8):18580-600.
2. Quesada E, Scott FB, Cardus D. Functional classification of neurogenic bladder dysfunction. Arch Phys Med Rehab. 1968;49:692-7.
3. Wein AJ. Classification of neurogenic voiding dysfunction. J Urol. 1981;125(5): 605-9.
4. Lapides J. Neuromuscular, vesical and ureteral dysfunction. In: Campbell MF, Harrison JH, editors. Urology. Philadelphia: Saunders; 1970. P. 1343-279.
5. Laycock J. What can the specialist physiotherapist do? In: Wyndaele JJ, Laycock J, eds. Multidisciplinary Conservative Treatment for the Neurogenic Bladder. Wokingham: Incare, 2002. P. 14-8.
6. Plevnik S, Homan G, Vrtacnik P. Short-term maximal electrical stimulation for urinary retention. Urology. 1984;24:521-3.
7. Ginsberg D. Optimizing therapy and management of neurogenic bladder. Am J Manag Care. 2013;19(Suppl 10):197-204.
8. Thavaseelan J. Botulinum toxin treatment for neurogenic detrusor overactivity. Incont Pelvic Floor Dysfunct. 2007;1:1-3.

9. Ginsberg D, Gousse A, Keppenne V, et al. Phase 3 efficacy and tolerability study of onabotulinumtoxinA for urinary incontinence from neurogenic detrusor overactivity. J Urol. 2012;187:2131-39.
10. Sakamoto K, Uvelius B, Khan T, et al. Preliminary study of a genetically engineered spinal cord implant on urinary bladder after experimental spinal cord injury in rats. J Rehabil Res Dev. 2002;39(3):347-57.
11. Park WB, Kim SY, Lee SH, et al. The effect of mesenchymal stem cell transplantation on the recovery of bladder and hindlimb function after spinal cord contusion in rats. BMC Neurosci. 2010;11:119.
12. Lima C, Escada P, Pratas-Vital J, et al. Olfactory mucosal autografts and rehabilitation for chronic traumatic spinal cord injury. Neurorehabil Neural Repair. 2010;24(1):10-22.
13. Groen J, Pannek J, Castro Diaz D, Del Popolo G, et al. Summary of European Association of Urology (EAU) Guidelines on Neuro-Urology. European Urology. 2016;69(2):324-33.

CHAPTER 2

Clinical Approach to Carpal Tunnel Syndrome

Bhanu Kesavamurthy, Senthil Nathan

INTRODUCTION

Carpal tunnel syndrome (CTS) is defined as a "constellation of clinical symptoms and signs caused by compression and slowing of median nerve at the wrist".[1] It is the most common entrapment neuropathy encountered in neurological practice.[2] It usually presents with mild to severe pain in hand especially at night, common among females, diabetic patients and in hypothyroid and pregnant. Though objective sensory and motor finding are rare, it causes severe disturbances in performing routine activities of daily living.

PATHOPHYSIOLOGY

Carpal tunnel syndrome is due to compression of median nerve at the carpal tunnel at wrist (Fig. 1). Carpal tunnel is a hollow tunnel formed by tubercles of scaphoid and trapezium radially and pisiform and hook of hamate carpal bones medially, forming the floor and transverse carpal ligament forming roof (Fig. 2). The exact mechanism of compression is not clear but mechanical injury seems to play an important role. The median nerve is compressed in closed space (carpel tunnel) by surrounding tissue or increase in interstitial fluid pressure[3]. Other causes includes neoplasm, infiltrative disease, infection, arthritis, deformities, and fracture of carpal bones. It is also common among diabetic patients and patients with hypothyroidism (Box 1). Some occupations that require constant wrist movement also resulted in CTS.[4]

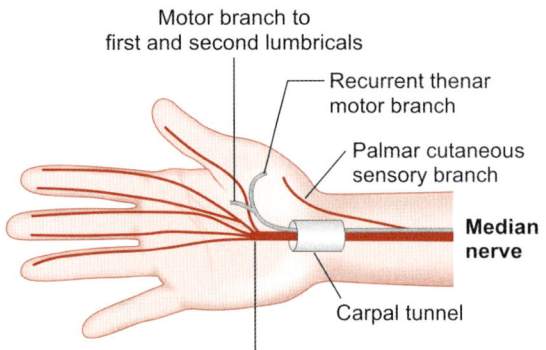

FIG. 1: Surface anatomy of carpal tunnel.

FIG. 2: Cross sectional anatomy of carpal tunnel.

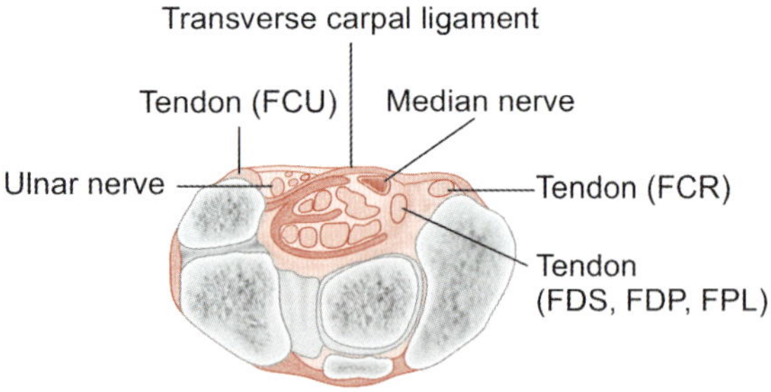

FCU, flexor carpi ulnaris; FCR, flexor carpi radialis; FDS, flexor digitorum superficialis; FDP, flexor digitorum profundus; FPL, flexor pollicis longus.

Compression of nerve results in reduced epineural blood flow, impairing axonal transport resulting in intraneural vascular injury due to increased pressure and endoneural edema. These changes lead to conduction block and ectopic impulse production which causes pain and numbness (Box 2).[3]

Box 1: Disorders associated with the carpal tunnel syndrome

- Amyloidosis
- Carpal tunnel lipoma
- Collagen disease
- Diabetes mellitus
- Dyschondroplasia
- Ganglion
- Gout
- Herpes zoster
- Hodgkin's disease
- Leukaemia
- Median artery thrombosis
- Mononeuritis multiplex
- Multiple myeloma
- Multiple sclerosis
- Neurofibromatosis
- Peripheral neuropathy
- Plantar fasciitis
- Polycythaemia
- Raynaud's phenomenon
- Renal failure
- Sarcoidosis
- Tuberculosis

Box 2: Neurological differential diagnoses[4]

- Congenital thenar hypoplasia
- Proximal median neuropathy
- Ulnar neuropathy
- Radial neuropathy
- Peripheral neuropathy
- Brachial plexopathy
- Thoracic outlet syndrome
- Cervical radiculopathy
- Motor neuron disease
- Syringomyelia
- Myelopathy

Box 3: Clinical features highly suggestive of carpal tunnel syndrome

- Nocturnal paresthesias sometimes awakening patient from sleep
- Pain and paresthesia brought on by driving or holding a book or newspaper
- Sensory disturbance in tips of first three digits and splitting the 4th digit
- Phalen's maneuver reproduces pain and paresthesias
- Weakness/wasting of thenar eminence

Box 4: Clinical features suggestive possible carpal tunnel syndrome

- Hand, wrist, forearm, arm, and/or shoulder pain
- Paresthesias involving all five digits
- No fixed sensory disturbance
- Decreased hand dexterity
- Tinel's sign over the median nerve at the wrist

Box 5: Clinical features inconsistent with carpal tunnel syndrome

- Neck pain
- Paresthesias and no pain
- Unequivocal numbness over the thenar eminence
- Weakness/wasting of hypothenar muscles
- Reduced biceps or triceps reflexes

CLINICAL FEATURES

Patient presents intermittent numbness, pain and paresthesia in the region in innervated by the median nerve. Symptoms are more severe in night, often awakening patients from sleep and is relieved by shaking or wringing hand. In severe cases patients notice weakness on prolonged hand grip, which improves with rest.[5] Thenar weakness and wasting seen in severe cases. Carpal tunnel syndrome is mostly unilaterally affecting dominant hand but it can also occur bilaterally.[6] Uncommon presentations includes palm and finger swelling and stiffness and loss of dexterity, painless thenar muscle wasting. Very rare presentations includes ulceration of the tips of index and middle finger and acroparesthesias of all finger (Boxes 3 to 5). A number of provocative test are used in clinical diagnosis of CTS, which are listed in table. Most commonly used test are Phalen's test and Tinel's sign but their accuracy in diagnosing CTS is still debatable (Table 1).[7]

There are various clinical scoring questionnaires to diagnose and assess severity of CTS. A scored questionnaire can replace nerve conduction studies in the initial assessment of patients presenting with CTS. The widely used questionnaire is based on the work of Levine et al. The questionnaire has been validated in secondary care for the diagnosis of CTS by Kamath et al.

Table 1: Clinical signs in carpal tunnel syndrome	
Test	Definition of abnormal finding[7]
Closed-fist sign	Paraesthesia in the distribution of the median nerve with the patient maintaining fist closure for 60 s
Flick sign	The patient demonstrates a flicking movement of the wrist and hand when describing their attempts to relieve their symptoms
Hand elevation test	Symptoms occur when patients raise their hands over their heads for up to 2 min
Phalen's test	Paresthesia in the distribution of the median nerve on sustained flexion of both wrists at 90° for 60 s
Pressure provocation test	Paresthesia in the distribution of the median nerve when the examiner presses with their thumb on the palmar aspect of the patient's wrist at the level of the carpal tunnel for 60 s
Square wrist	Wrist ratio >0.70. The wrist ratio is the anteroposterior dimension of the wrist divided by the mediolateral dimension (measured at the distal flexor crease)
Tinel's sign	Tapping the distal wrist crease over the median nerve results in paresthesia in the distribution of the median nerve

Table 2: A neurophysiological system for grading the severity of the carpal tunnel syndrome[9]	
Grade 0	Normal
Grade 1	Very mild, abnormal nerve conduction only demonstrable with most sensitive tests
Grade 2	Mild, sensory nerve conduction velocity slowing, and normal terminal median nerve motor latency
Grade 3	Moderate, preserved sensory action potentials, and distal motor latency <6.5 ms
Grade 4	Severe, absent sensory action potentials, and distal motor latency <6.5 ms
Grade 5	Very severe, distal motor latency >6.5 ms
Grade 6	Extremely severe; unrecordable sensory and motor action potentials

INVESTIGATIONS

Electrophysiological testing is the main stay in diagnosing CTS, other than clinical means. Electrophysiological test helps to confirm distal median neuropathy, grade CTS and to rule out other causes. Standard tests used are distal median motor latency, antidromic sensory recording from median nerve and variety of Internal Comparison test like median-ulnar palm-wrist mixed nerve studies, median versus ulnar wrist to digit 4 sensory latency study, median versus radial digit 1 sensory latency, and median second lumbrical versus ulnar interossei distal motor latency.[8] Other electrodiagnostic tests include inching technique and terminal latency index. Sensory nerves are more susceptible injury and ischemia. Hence sensory nerve conduction studies are involved earlier in the course of disease (Table 2).

Electrophysiological Tests[10]

Distal Median Motor Latency

Recording is done from the abductor pollicis brevis while the median nerve is stimulated 3 cm proximal to distal crease of the wrist. Onset latency greater than 4.2 ms, and compound muscle action potential (CMAP) amplitude less than 5 mV and difference between both hand latency greater than 0.7 ms is considered abnormal.[10] Specificity of the abnormal values greater than 4.2 was 99%.

Antidromic Sensory Recording From Median Nerve

Recording ring electrodes are placed over the 2nd digit with active electrode over the proximal phalanx and reference over the distal part of middle phalanx. The median nerve is stimulated 13 cm proximal to the active electrode just above the wrist. At this location median nerve runs between the flexor carpi radialis tendon radially and the palmaris longus tendon medially.

Normal values are distal latency less than 3.5 ms, amplitude greater than 15 mV, conduction velocity greater than 56 m/s.

Prolongation of peak latency greater than 3.5 ms and peak-to-peak amplitude of sensory nerve action potential less than 10 μV and right-left latency difference greater than 0.5 ms are considered abnormal.[8]

Median-Ulnar Palm-Wrist Mixed Nerve Studies

This test is done by stimulating both motor and sensory component of nerve. This test includes large myelinated fires which are more susceptible to demyelination. The median recording electrode is placed proximal to the wrist crease, overlies the median nerve between the flexor carpi radialis and palmaris longus tendons. The ulnar electrode is placed proximal to the wrist crease just medial of the flexor carpi ulnaris tendon. The reference electrodes are placed 3.5–4.0 cm proximal to active electrodes. The normal values are distal latency less than 2.3 ms, amplitude greater than 50 mV, conduction velocity greater than 56 m/s for median nerve and distal latency less than 2.3 ms, amplitude greater than 15 mV, conduction velocity greater than 55 m/s for ulnar nerve. The difference between median and ulnar latency is 0.3 ms or less. A latency difference greater than 0.4 ms is considered significant.[11]

Median Versus Ulnar Wrist to Digit 4 Sensory Latency Study

Here median and ulnar nerve are stimulated at wrist and sensory potential at 4th digit measured (as it has dual innervation). Median sensory latency greater than 3.5 ms or difference in latency between median and ulnar greater than 0.5 ms is considered as significant.[11]

Median Versus Radial Digit 1 Sensory Latency

In this test median nerve is compared with radial nerve. Ring electrodes are placed over thumb. The median and radial nerves are stimulated above the wrist at a distance of 10 cm proximal to the proximal ring electrode. The distances must be identical. Difference in latency greater than 0.5 ms is considered abnormal.[12]

Median Second Lumbrical Versus Ulnar Interossei Distal Motor Latency

This is the only test where motor studies are used. In this study, the median motor latency recording the second lumbrical is compared to the ulnar latency recording the interossei, using identical distances between stimulation and recording sites. Difference in latency greater than 0.5 ms is considered abnormal. It is used when all sensory responses are absent and also in extreme CTS as these fibers are most resistant and are affected last.[11]

Inching Technique

This technique is also useful in demonstrating CTS. It was first described by Kimura et al. Median nerve is stimulated sequentially at a distance of 1 cm, a sudden drop in amplitude and increase in latency cross wrist is highly suggestive of CTS. However, this test has high false positive results and should be read with caution.[13]

Terminal Latency Index

It adjusts the distal latency for terminal distance and proximal nerve conduction velocity.[13]

$$\frac{\text{Terminal distance (mm)}}{\text{Conduction velocity (ms)} \times \text{Terminal latency (ms)}}$$

Needle Electromyography

Electromyography (EMG) helps in identifying chronic denervation of muscles. Carpal tunnel syndrome is characterized by involvement of only abductor pollicis brevis. Presence of denervation of muscles other than abductor pollicis brevis is characterized of other causes like flexor carpi radialis (Proximal median lesion), pronator teres, triceps (C6-C7 radiculopathy) (Boxes 6 to 9).

Ultrasonography

High resolution sonography is now an emerging tool in diagnosing CTS. Transducers at frequency of 7–12 MHz is used to study median nerve. The cross sectional area of the median nerve is measured at multiple levels especially

Box 6: Recommended nerve conduction study protocol for carpal tunnel syndrome

Routine studies:
- Median motor study recording abductor pollicis brevis, stimulating wrist and antecubital fossa
- Ulnar motor study recording abductor digiti minimi, stimulating wrist, below groove, and above groove
- Median and ulnar F responses
- Median sensory response, recording digit 2 or 3, stimulating wrist
- Ulnar sensory response, recording digit 5, stimulating wrist

Median vs. ulnar comparisons:
- Comparison of the median and ulnar mixed palm-to-wrist peak latencies
- Comparison of the median lumbrical and ulnar interossei distal motor latencies, stimulating the median and ulnar wrist one at a time at identical distances
- Comparison of the median and ulnar digit 4 sensory latencies, stimulating the median and ulnar wrist one at a time at identical distances

Median inching across the wrist:
- Motor inching across the wrist into the palm at 1-cm intervals looking for an abrupt change in latency (>0.3 ms) or significant increase in CMAP amplitude (distal/proximal ratio >1.2)
- Sensory inching across the wrist into the palm at 1-cm intervals looking for an abrupt change in latency (>0.3 ms) or significant increase in SNAP amplitude (distal/proximal ratio >1.6)

CMAP, compound muscle action potential; SNAP, sensory nerve action potential.

Box 7: Electrophysiological features suggestive of carpal tunnel syndrome

- The routine studies of median nerve showing marked slowing across the wrist in the form of prolonged distal motor, sensory latencies, and prolonged minimum F wave latencies (amplitudes may be diminished if there is secondary axonal loss or conduction block at the wrist)
- The ulnar motor, sensory, and F wave studies are normal
- If two or three of the median vs. ulnar comparison tests or the inching studies are abnormal

Box 8: Electrophysiological differential diagnosis of carpal tunnel syndrome

If they do localize to the wrist-
- Carpal tunnel syndrome with coexistent ulnar neuropathy at the elbow
- Carpal tunnel syndrome and a coexistent polyneuropathy resulting in ulnar abnormalities
- Carpal tunnel syndrome and a brachial plexopathy

If they do not localize to the wrist—more diffuse abnormality
- Brachial plexopathy or a polyneuropathy

Box 9: Recommended electromyographic protocol for Carpal tunnel syndrome

- Abductor pollicis brevis (APB)
- At least two C6-C7 muscles to exclude a cervical radiculopathy (e.g., pronator teres, triceps brachii, and extensor digitorum communis)
- At least one proximal median muscle to exclude a proximal median neuropathy (e.g., flexor carpi radialis, pronator teres, and flexor pollicis longus)
- At least two other nonmedian, lower trunk C8–T1 muscles, to exclude a lower trunk brachial plexopathy, polyneuropathy, or C8–T1 radiculopathy (e.g., first dorsal interosseous, extensor indicis proprius)

at inlet and outlet for carpal tunnel. Thickening of nerve is considered as sign of inflammation of the nerve. It also helps to visualize nerve fascicles (Fig. 3).[14]

Magnetic Resonance Imaging

Magnetic resonance imaging (MRI) of median nerve can be used to demonstrate abnormalities like swelling or flattering of median nerve. Hyperintensity of nerve signaling and bowing of flexor retinaculum are the typical finding seen in MRI in patients with CTS.[15]

MANAGEMENT

Main objectives of treating CTS are relief of sensory symptoms, prevent progression, limit disability and maximize functional capacity. Conservative management includes splinting, medication, and intracarpal steroid injections.

Clinical Approach to Carpal Tunnel Syndrome

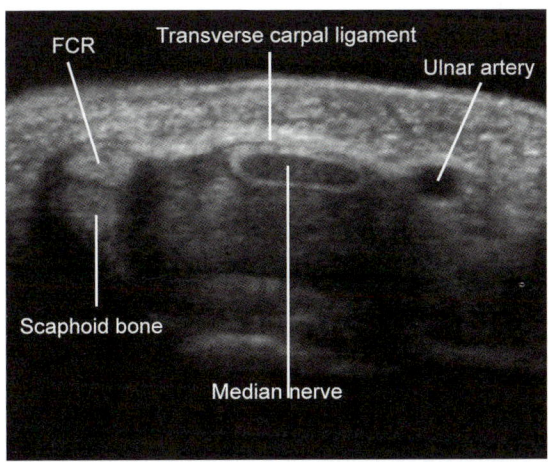

FIG. 3: Ultrasound in carpal tunnel syndrome.

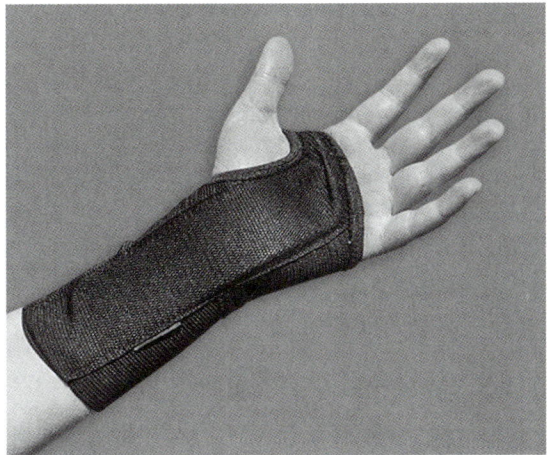

FIG. 4: Splinting. *(For color version, see Plate 1)*

When conservative management fails patient is adviced surgical correction. Treatment of primary cause like rheumatoid arthritis, hypothyroidism relieves symptoms in the affected patients.

Splinting
Normal pressure in carpal tunnel is between 0 and 7 mm Hg which increases during wrist movement, flexion and extension. Splinting in neutral position with prefabricated splints has given effective relief in majority of patients and has even postponed the need for surgery in few cases. It has to be worn continuously to obtain better results (Fig. 4).[16,17]

Drug Treatment
Prednisolone in doses of 10–25 mg daily for 2 weeks appear to be effective for short-term improvement of CTS symptoms. Drugs used for neuropathy like gabapentin, pregabalin, and carbamazepine are used with little benefits. Other drugs tried in includes pyridoxine, diuretics, and nonsteroidal anti-inflammatory drugs, but results are not promising for future studies.

Intracarpal injection of corticosteroid has produced better results. It decreases the volume of the swollen tissue. It is injected on the ulnar side of the palmaris, beneath flexor retinaculum. The risk of median nerve injury limits this procedure. Other site is proximal to carpal tunnel where needle is inserted, 4 cm proximal to distal wrist increase. It gives better results but short lasting, recurrence common on long term. Various factors that are implicated in poor prognosis and recurrences are symptoms more than year, muscle wasting (thenar), nerve conduction study showing absent sensory nerve action potentials (SNAPs) and prolonged distal motor latencies (>6 cm).[18]

SURGERY
Indications for carpal tunnel release surgery include persistent numbness and pain, refractory to medical management and splinting, motor dysfunction like diminished grip or pinch grasping, or thenar wasting.

Before planning for surgical carpal tunnel release, the diagnosis of CTS should be confirmed clinically and electrophysiologically. Although, most common cause of median nerve entrapment at the wrist is CTS, other disorders, such as cervical radiculopathy, thoracic outlet syndrome and pronator syndrome must be ruled out.

The decompression of the nerve is done by splitting the transverse carpal ligament by opening carpal tunnel is the standard procedure done. Additionally intraoperative, internal neurolysis is done for better results. Here the nerve is divided into multiple fascicles. Endoscopic carpal tunnel release is a newer technique with better results and rapid recovery, is being done nowadays. The causes for relapse of symptoms after surgery includes, misdiagnosis, incomplete division of flexor retinaculum, nerve branch injury during procedure and perineural fibrosis (Fig. 5).[19]

Other lines of management includes ultrasound treatment which is believed to have anti-inflammatory effect and better nerve regeneration. Yoga, a course of 2–3 hours of workouts for 8 weeks seems to promote relief. Magnet therapy, chiropractic care, acupuncture, hydrotherapy, and massage has been tried, but no supporting data available.[20]

PROGNOSIS

Prognosis is usually better in milder forms, secondary to disease and those showing minimal changes in electrophysiology. Longer duration (>6 months), older age, alcohol use, muscle wasting, absent SNAP's and CMAP's and poor response to corticosteroid injection are the main factors for poor outcome and relapses.[21]

CONCLUSION

Carpal tunnel syndrome is the commonest entrapment neuropathy in clinical practice. It is more common among women and in dominant hand. Though diagnosis is made clinically variety of electrophysiological test available to confirm it. Treatment is mainly conservative with splinting, medicine, and intracarpal steroid injections. Those who do not respond to conservative treatment, who have relapses, muscle wasting may benefit from early surgery.

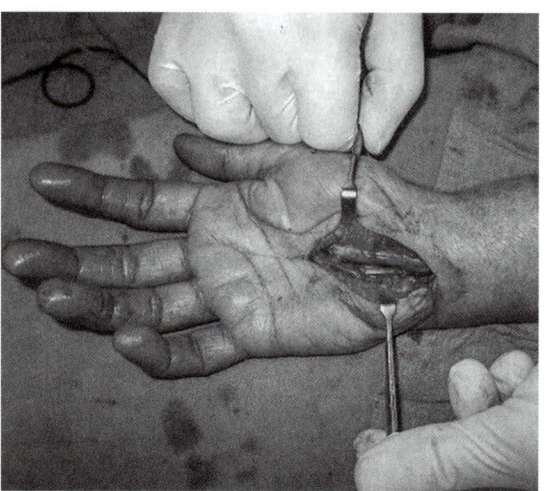

FIG. 5: Surgical decompression of carpal tunnel. *(For color version, see Plate 1)*

CASE VIGNETTES

CASE-1

A 58-year-old female presented with complaints of pain and tingling sensations in both hands for 7 months duration. Symptoms were worse at night and she had to get up from sleep at times with severe pain and numbness. Pain increased on lifting weight, washing utensils, and stitching clothes. On examination there was mild wasting of thenar eminence and sensory loss over finger pads on thumb, index finger and ring finger, and mild weakness of thumb abduction. Rest of examination were normal. On eliciting Phalen's maneuver, patient has pain in wrist, middle finger, and numbness over finger pads increased. Patient is a known case of type 2 diabetes mellitus under poor glycemic control.

Nerve Conduction Study

Table 5: Nerve conduction study values

Nerve stimulated	Stimulation site	Recording site	Amplitude		Latency		Conduction velocity		F-wave latency	
			R	L	R	L	R	L	R	L
Median (M)	Wrist	APB	3.3	8.8	10	6.6	43	49	38	34
	Elbow	APB	3.1	8.6	14	11	–	–	–	–

Clinical Approach to Carpal Tunnel Syndrome

Ulnar (M)	Wrist	ADM	11.4	11.2	3.1	3.2	60	61.2	25.2	24.8
	Elbow	ADM	11.2	11.1	6.1	6.4	–	–	–	–
Median (s)	Wrist	Index finger	2.8	8	5.8	4.9	28	32	–	–
Ulnar (s)	Wrist	Little finger	24	26	2.8	2.9	62	–	–	–
Median Mixed study	Palm	Wrist	NR	12	NR	4.2	NR	27	–	–
Ulnar Mixed study	Palm	Wrist	16	18	1.8	1.9	62	61	–	–

Electromyography

Muscle	Spontaneous activity			Voluntary motor unit action potentials				
	Insertional activity	Fibrillations	Fasciculations	Activation	Recruitment	Duration	Amplitude	Polyphasia
Rt APB	Increased	+1	0	NL	Decreased	+2	+2	+2
Rt FDI	NL	0	0	NL	NL	NL	NL	NL
Rt TRICEPS	NL	0	0	NL	NL	NL	NL	NL
Rt FCR	NL	0	0	NL	NL	NL	NL	NL
Rt PT	NL	0	0	NL	NL	NL	NL	NL
Lt APB	NL	0	0	NL	NL	NL	NL	NL

Table 6: Electromyography

APB, abductor pollicis brevis; ADM, abductor digiti minimi; FCR, flexor carpi radialis; FDI, first dorsal interosseous; PT, pronator teres.

Observations made with nerve conduction study (NCS) and EMG in this patient are:
- Median motor study on right hand shows decreased CMAP amplitude, prolonged distal latency, and slower conduction velocity. Prolonged F minimum latency
- Left median study also abnormal with prolonged distal latency, moderate slowing of conduction velocity and prolonged F minimum latency. However CMAP amplitude is normal
- Median sensory on both sides abnormal with increased distal latency and show conduction velocity
- Ulnar motor and sensory studies were normal on both sides (which excludes widespread polyneuropathy or radiculopathy)
- Median sensory response to digit 2 absent on right but present with low amplitude prolonged distal latency and slower conduction velocity in right
- The median mixed latency is prolonged out of proportion to ulnar mixed peak latency
- Electromyography showed denervation changes in right abductor pollicis brevis (APB) but normal responses in pronator teres (PT) and flexor carpi radialis (FCR), indicating the lesson in median nerve is restricted only to distal portion whereas proximally supplied muscles are spared. It also rules out cervical radiculopathy (C6–C7)
- Since APB was normal in left other muscles were not tested.

The NCS and EMG features in this case were suggestive of bilateral moderately severe median neuropathy are wrist (right greater than left).

CASE-2

A 49-year-old female, diagnosed as rheumatoid arthritis 6 months ago, presented with complaints of pain and paresthesia for past 2 months. Symptoms were worse at night awakening her from sleep, twice sometimes and she had shake and press her hand to get relieved. Activities like holding book, telephone, and driving bikes worsens the pain. On clinical examination there was mild decreased in touch sensation over finger pads of middle and index finger on right and rest of routine neurological examination was normal. Phalen's maneuver elicited paresthesia after 60 seconds.

Table 7: Nerve conduction study

Nerve stimulated	Stimulation site	Recording site	Amplitude		Latency		Conduction velocity		F-Wave latency	
			R	L	R	L	R	L	R	L
Median (M)	Wrist	APB	6.2	6.1	4.2	4.1	58	56	29	28
	Elbow	APB	6.0	6.0	7.9	7.6	–	–	–	–
Ulnar (M)	Wrist	ADM	9.0	8.8	2.9	2.8	57	58	28	27
	Elbow	ADM	8.9	8.6	6.4	6.4	–	–	–	–
Median (s)	Wrist	Index finger	24	26	3.3	3.2	56	58	–	–
Ulnar (s)	Wrist	Little finger	23	26	2.9	2.7	62	60	–	–
Median Mixed study	Palm	Wrist	30 N >50	54	2.4 N <2.2	2.1	40 N>50	55	–	–
Ulnar Mixed study	Palm	Wrist	15 N >12	16	1.8 N <2.2	1.9	62 N >50	60	–	–
Mixed difference	–		0.6		N <0.3		–		–	–
Median lumbrical	Wrist	Second lumbrical	1.4 N >1.0	1.6	3.7	–	–	–	–	–
Ulnar	Wrist	Interossei	4.5 N >2.5	4.6	2.9	–	–	–	–	–
Lumbrical-Interossei difference			0.8		N <0.4		–		–	–
Median (s)	Wrist	Ring finger	21 N >10		3.4		40 N >50	–	–	–
Ulnar (s)	Wrist	Ring finger	23 N >10		2.8		52 N >50	–	–	–
Digit 4 difference			0.6		N <0.4		–	–	–	–

Nerve conduction studies and EMG findings:
- NCS shows normal median and ulnar motor and sensory conduction studies
- However following findings point to carpal tunnel syndrome
- The median versus ulnar, palm to wrist latency difference is 0.6 ms. (normal <0.4 ms)
- The comparison of median lumbrical and ulnar interossei distal motor latency is 0.8 ms. (normal <0.5 ms)
- Comparison of median and ulnar digit 4 sensory latencies showed a difference of 0.6ms (normal <0.5 ms)

Though routine nerve conduction studies were normal, median versus ulnar comparison studies favoured CTS, hence patient was diagnosed as CTS and treated accordingly.

Table 8: Electromyography

Muscle	Spontaneous activity			Voluntary motor unit action potentials				
	Insertional activity	Fibrillations	Fasciculations	Activation	Recruitment	Duration	Amplitude	Polyphasia
Rt APB	NL	0	0	NL	NL	NL	NL	NL
Rt FDI	NL	0	0	NL	NL	NL	NL	NL
Rt TRICEPS	NL	0	0	NL	NL	NL	NL	NL
Rt FCR	NL	0	0	NL	NL	NL	NL	NL
Rt PT	NL	0	0	NL	NL	NL	NL	NL

APB, abductor pollicis brevis; FCR, flexor carpi radialis; PT, pronator teres; FDI, first dorsal interosseous.

REFERENCES

1. Phalen GS. The carpal tunnel syndrome. Seventeen years experience in diagnosis and treatment of six hundred fifty – four hands. J Bone Joint Surg. 1996;48:211-28.
2. Atroshi I, Gummesson C, Johnsson R, et al. Prevalence of carpal tunnel syndrome in a general population. JAMA. 1999;28:2153-8.
3. Werner RA, Andary M. Carpal tunnel syndrome: Pathophysiology and clinical neurophysiology. Review. Clin Neurophysiol. 2002;113:1373-81.
4. Rosenbaum RB, Ochoa JC. Carpal Tunnel Syndrome and Other Disorders of the Median Nerve, 2nd edn. Butterworth-Heinemann, Woburn. 2002.
5. [No authors listed]. Practice parameter for carpal tunnel syndrome (summary statement). Report of the Quality Standards Subcommittee of the American Academy of Neurology. Neurology. 1993;43:2406-9.
6. Bland JD, Rudolfer SM. Clinical surveillance of carpal tunnel syndrome in two areas of the United Kingdom, 1991–2001. J Neurol Neurosurg Psychiatry. 2003;74(12):1674-9.
7. D'Arcy CA, McGee S. Does this patient have carpal tunnel syndrome? JAMA. 2000;283:3110-7.
8. American Association of Electrodiagnostic Medicine. American Academy of Neurology. American Academy of Physical Medicine and Rehabilitation Practice parameter: Electrodiagnostic studies in carpal tunnel syndrome. Neurology. 2002;58:1589-92.
9. Padua L, LoMonaco M, Gregori B, et al. Neurophysiological classification and sensitivity in 500 carpal tunnel syndrome hands. Acta Neurol Scand. 1997;96:211-7.
10. Padua L, Lo Monaco M, Valento EM, et al. A useful electrophysiologic parameter for diagnosis of carpal tunnel syndrome. Muscle Nerve. 1996;19:48-53.
11. Uncini A, Di Muzio A, Awad J, et al. Sensitivity of three median-to-ulnar comparative tests in diagnosis of mild carpal tunnel syndrome. Muscle Nerve. 1993;16:1366-73.
12. Carroll GJ. Comparison of median and radial nerve sensory latencies in the electrophysiological diagnosis of carpal tunnel syndrome. Electroencephalogr Clin Neurophysiol. 1987;68:101-6
13. Kimura J. The carpal tunnel syndrome: Localization of conduction abnormalities within the distal segment of the median nerve. Brain. 1979;102:619-35.
14. Ziswiler HR, Reichenbach S, Vogelin E, et al. Diagnostic value of sonography in patients with suspected carpal tunnel syndrome: A prospective study. Arthritis Rheum. 2005;52:304-11.
15. Jarvik JG, Yuen E, Haynor DR et al. MR nerve imaging in a prospective cohort of patients with suspected carpal tunnel syndrome. Neurology. 2002;58:1597-602.
16. Gelberman RH, Aronson D, Weisman MH. Carpal tunnel syndrome Results of a prospective trial of steroid injection and splinting. J Bone Joint Surg Am. 1980;62(7):1181-4.
17. Gerritsen AA, de Vet H, Sholten RJ, et al. Splinting vs. surgery in the treatment of carpal tunnel syndrome. JAMA. 2002;288:1245-51.
18. Ozdogan H, Yazici H. The efficacy of local steroid injections in idiopathic carpal tunnel syndrome: A double-blind study. Br J Rheumatol. 1984;23:272-5.
19. Scholten RJPM, Gerritsen AAM, Uitdehaag BMJ, et al. Surgical treatment options for carpal tunnel syndrome. The Cochrane Database of Systematic Reviews. 2004;4:CD003905.
20. O'Connor D, Marshall S, Massy-Westropp N. Non-surgical treatment (other than steroid injection) for carpal tunnel syndrome. Cochrane Database Systematic Reviews. 2003;1:CD003219.
21. Finestone HM, Woodbury GM, Collavini T, et al. Severe carpal tunnel syndrome. Clinical and electrodiagnostic outcome of surgical and conservative treatment. Muscle and Nerve. 1996;19:237-9.

CHAPTER 3

Bidirectional Interaction Between Sleep and Epilepsy: Practice Points

Athi Ponnusamy

INTRODUCTION

The interaction between sleep and epilepsy is bidirectional and is well known for centuries. In 350 BC, Aristotle noted the connections between epilepsy and sleep.[1] Gowers has documented in his treatise about the timing of seizure occurrence in relationship to the sleep-wake cycle.[2] With similar clinical observation, Langdon and Brain have identified diurnal epilepsy in 1929.[3] In the same year, Berger has recorded electroencephalogram in humans. Gibbs and Gibbs in 1947 documented the fact that interictal epileptiform discharges are enhanced in sleep in people with epilepsy.[4]

The relationship between sleep and epilepsy are complex. Each affect adversely the other to reduce the quality of life (QoL), increase morbidity and possibly sudden unexpected death in epilepsy (SUDEP). Sleep has an important role in memory consolidation and reinforcement.[5] Sleep is also essential for restoration of various physiological homeostatic processes and synaptic integrity. Sleep deprivation impairs these vital body functions and epilepsy due to nocturnal seizures can upset these vital processes. Sleep disorders are up to three times as common in people with epilepsy and can be a major trigger for refractory seizures and high morbidity.[6] Prompt diagnosis and successful treatment of both epilepsy and sleep disorders lead to better outcomes and QoL in patients. In this review, the bidirectional interaction between epilepsy and sleep have been highlighted.

IMPACT OF SLEEP/SLEEP DEPRIVATION ON EPILEPSY

Nonrapid eye movement (NREM) sleep has been described as a physiologic state of relative neuronal synchronization, which facilitates the recruitment of the critical mass of neurons needed to initiate and sustain a seizure. Generalized spike wave discharges preferentially occur during NREM sleep, particularly during the lighter stages when sleep spindles are present.[7] Hence, seizures occur more frequently in NREM sleep compared with rapid eye movement (REM) sleep or awake state. Focal seizures from frontal lobe networks occur predominantly during NREM sleep. Seizures during sleep are more likely to secondarily generalize.

Sleep deprivation is a common trigger for seizure occurrence in many patients. In animal research, it was found that cats are more susceptible to kindled and penicillin-induced seizures after sleep deprivation.[8] Total sleep deprivation increases the rate of kindling in the amygdala.[9] Transcranial magnetic stimulation found reduced short intracortical inhibition and increased intracortical facilitation in healthy volunteers after 24 hours of sleep deprivation.[10] These findings support increased cortical excitability. Sleep deprivation usually partial sleep deprivation is used as an activation procedure to facilitate seizure capture during video telemetry monitoring for diagnostic and presurgical evaluation. Both generalized seizures and of focal seizures are triggered after sleep deprivation. Sleep deprivation is often associated with an increase in interictal epileptiform discharges (Fig. 1) and poorer epilepsy control.

Epilepsy Syndromes Where Seizures are Potentiated During Sleep[5]

Focal Epilepsy Syndromes
- Benign childhood epilepsy with centro-temporal spikes (rolandic epilepsy) (Fig. 2)
- Benign childhood epilepsy with occipital paroxysm (Panayiotopoulos syndrome)
- Autosomal dominant nocturnal frontal lobe epilepsy (ADNFLE)
- Nocturnal frontal lobe epilepsy (NFLE)
- Nocturnal temporal lobe epilepsy.

Genetic Generalized Epilepsy Syndromes
- Juvenile myoclonic epilepsy (JME)
- Generalized tonic and clonic seizures on awakening.

Epileptic Encephalopathies in Children
- Epileptic encephalopathy with continuous spike and wave during slow wave sleep (CSWS) (Fig. 3)
- Landau–Kleffner syndrome (Acquired epileptic aphasia).

Paroxysmal Attacks in Sleep (Diagnostic Challenges)

Abnormal paroxysmal motor events in sleep poses a significant challenge for the clinician. These include parasomnias such as NREM parasomnias (sleepwalking, sleep terrors, and confusional arousals), REM parasomnias, movement disorders in sleep, epileptic seizures (Fig. 4), particularly in case of frontal lobe seizures (Fig. 5), and psychogenic nonepileptic attacks from pseudo-sleep. Each has different management plan and prognosis. Hence, correct diagnosis is paramount. In many cases, distinguishing seizures and parasomnias with careful and skillful clinical history is relatively straightforward. However, a diagnostic video-telemetry to analysis the clinical semiology of the paroxysmal events and time-locked ictal electroencephalography (EEG) will be helpful in difficult cases. Frontal lobe seizures present a particular difficulty as ictal scalp EEG may be normal and semiology of the attacks in the video data will be very helpful to clinch the diagnosis and proceed to further imaging and genetic investigations. Nocturnal frontal lobe epilepsy occurs sporadically or as an autosomal dominant inheritance. Autosomal dominant nocturnal frontal lobe epilepsy (ADNFLE) may

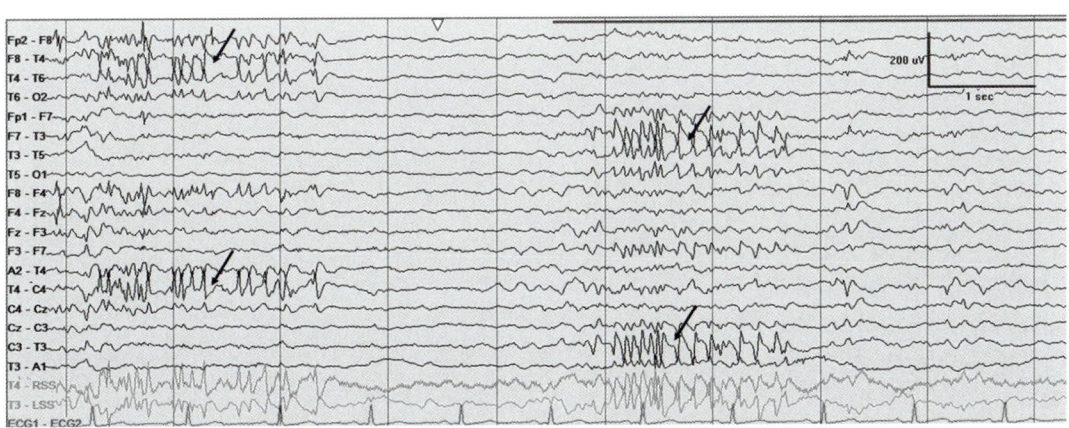

FIG. 1: Potentiation of spike wave discharges over temporal regions independently in slow wave sleep in a case of bitemporal temporal lobe epilepsy. *(For color version, see Plate 1)*

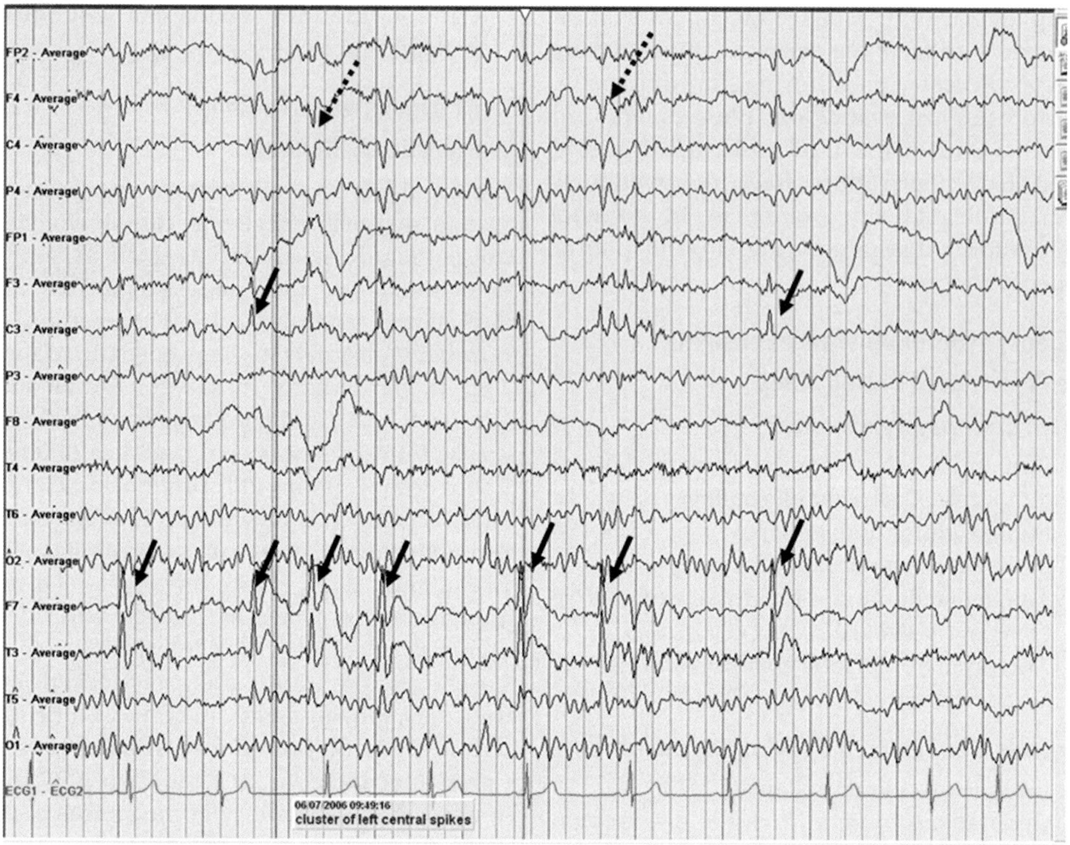

FIG. 2: Centro temporal spikes in a child with benign Rolandic epilepsy: Black arrows and dotted arrows highlight the negative spikes in centro temporal electrodes and positive spikes in frontal electrodes in common average derivation. *(For color version, see Plate 2)*

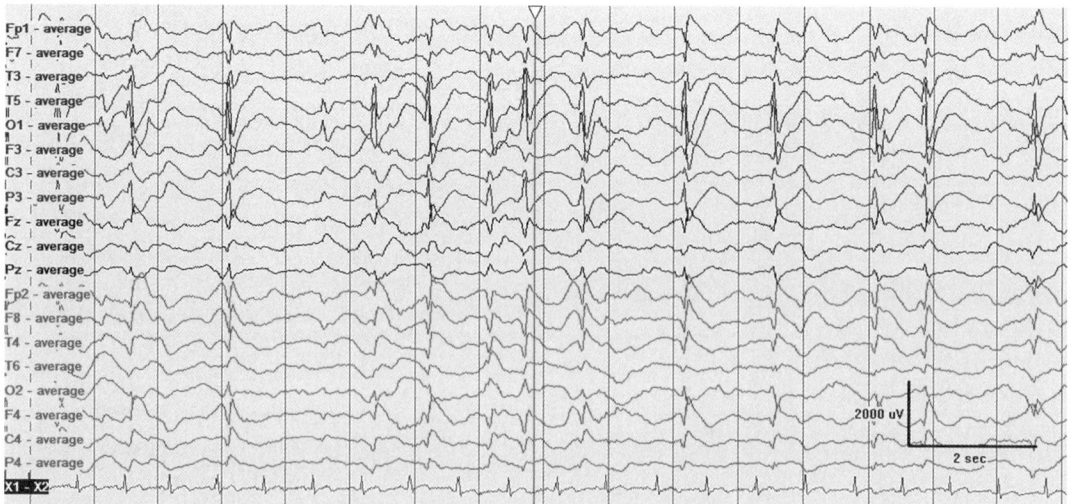

FIG. 3: Electrical status in slow wave sleep. If clinical features support global cognitive decline, diagnosis of continuous spike in slow wave sleep is diagnosed. *(For color version, see Plate 2)*

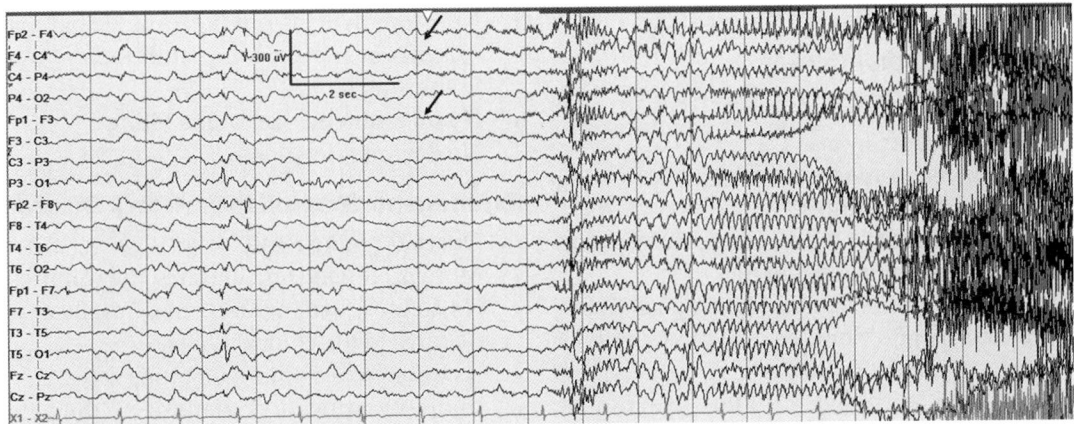

FIG. 4: Ictal scalp electroencephalography in a patient with genetic generalized epilepsy during one generalized tonic clonic seizure from slow-wave sleep. Black arrow corresponds to ictal onset with subsequent classic ictal evolution. *(For color version, see Plate 3)*

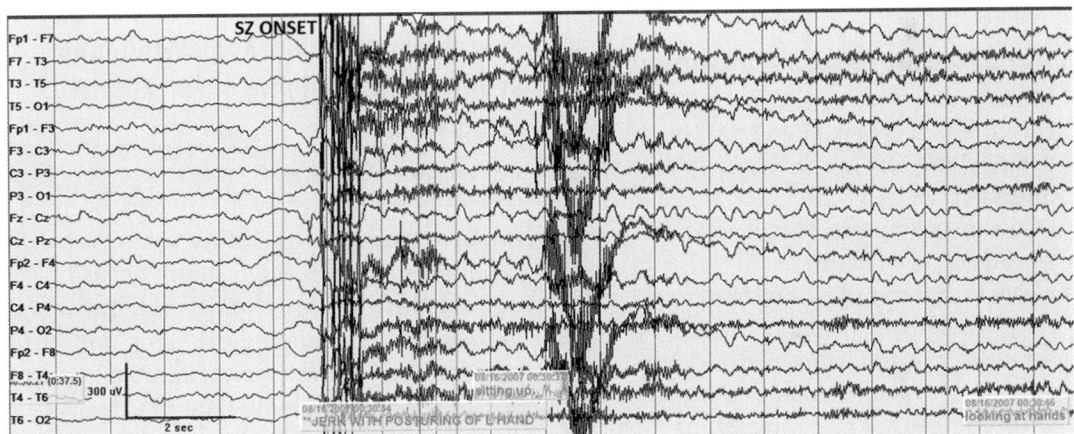

FIG. 5: Ictal scalp electroencephalography in a patient with nocturnal frontal lobe seizure during one brief clonic with asymmetric tonic seizure from slow-wave sleep. Note nonlocalized and nonlateralized ictal scalp electroencephalography pattern. (Semiology in video may be useful for localization and lateralization). *(For color version, see Plate 3)*

have bizarre complex motor features with or without vocalization and both EEG and magnetic resonance imaging (MRI) are unhelpful. This leads on to misdiagnosis and often these are labelled incorrectly as parasomnias or psychogenic seizures.

Derry et al. produced a clinical tool "Frontal lobe epilepsy and parasomnia (FLEP) scale" which was shown to differentiate nocturnal frontal lobe seizures from other sleep disorders with a diagnostic accuracy up to 94%.[11] This scale is based on salient clinical features seen in NFLE and parasomnia and each of the clinical feature is given a score and it comprises of 11 clinical features and a total composite score is taken to differentiate NFLE versus parasomnia. A score of zero or less in FLEP scale makes epilepsy very unlikely and a score of more than 3 makes epilepsy very likely and patients with a score between 1 and 3 need further investigation such as in-patient video-telemetry monitoring.

Clinical Pointers Helpful to Differentiate Paroxysmal Attacks in Sleep[5]

Epilepsy

- Age of onset at any age
- Stereotyped behavior in the attacks lasting for seconds to minutes
- Multiple attacks in the same night sleep; can occur at any time of the night
- Complex automatisms, posturing, head and eye version, and clonic jerks in the semiology
- Mostly amnesiac to events
- May have excessive daytime sleepiness (EDS)
- Incontinence, tongue bite, and injuries more common
- Will not leave the bed
- Will not have complex behavior like eating, talking, acting out, or intercourse.

Nonrapid Eye Movement Parasomnia

- Childhood onset
- No stereotyped behavior in the attacks
- Attacks last for many minutes (up to 30 minutes)
- One or two attacks in a night and often within 2 hours of onset of sleep
- Absence of complex automatisms, posturing, head and eye version, clonic jerks in the semiology; mostly amnesiac to events
- May have EDS particularly when associated with Periodic limb movement disorder (PLMD) or obstructive sleep apnea (OSA)
- Incontinence and tongue bite do not occur; injuries are very rare
- Usually will leave the bed and can have complex behavior like eating, talking, or rarely intercourse.

Rapid Eye Movement Parasomnia

- Onset during middle age or elderly
- Male predominance
- May not be aware; but if present can be distressing
- Dream enacting behavior present and if violent injuries can occur
- Can be multiple during a night; last for seconds and always start >4 hours after sleep onset
- Not stereotypical and no complex behavior
- Absence of version, tonic, and clonic features in the attack
- No incontinence or tongue biting
- No daytime sleepiness.

Psychogenic Nonepileptic Attack Disorder

- Onset as young adult
- More prolonged and at times >30 minutes
- No stereotypical nature; erratic and variable features in the clinical attacks
- Incontinence and tongue biting rare
- Injuries may occur depending on the nature of the attacks
- Can occur at any time of night
- May lead on to daytime sleepiness
- History of stressful life events, post-traumatic stress, and childhood sexual abuse.

Role of Diagnostic Video EEG Monitoring in Differential Diagnosis of Paroxysmal Attacks in Sleep

In nocturnal epileptic seizures, video of the attacks helps to classify the attacks as epileptic seizures and also to differentiate focal and generalized seizures. On many occasions, we will be able to localize and lateralize the seizures depending on semiological signs and aura if present. This review does not address this aspect of epileptology in detail. Ictal EEG has specific pattern to help us classify the seizures. Both video and EEG data are useful to differentiate epilepsy and parasomnia and psychogenic nonepileptic seizures. It is to be noted that in NFLE, ictal EEG may be normal, and semiology of the attack seen in the video is the most helpful for diagnosis. At times, postictal EEG abnormality is key to differentiate epileptic seizure and other nonepileptic events.

In parasomnia, the ictal and postictal EEG is normal with no epileptic rhythm and the EEG is helpful to know whether the parasomnia arise from slow-wave sleep (SWS) or REM sleep. Video data is also helpful to characterize the clinical features of the parasomnia. If the diagnostic video telemetry is done as a part of polysomnography (PSG) with electromyogram

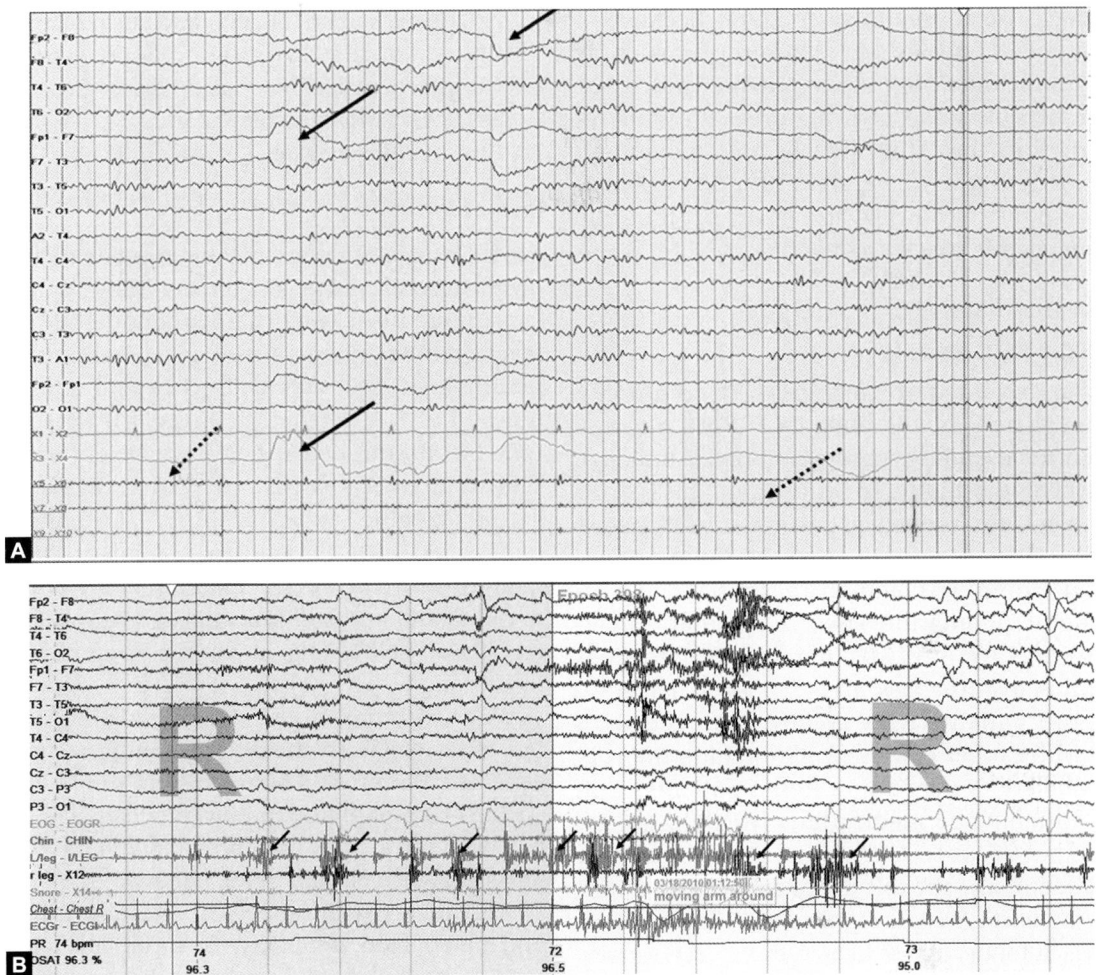

FIG. 6: A, Electroencephalography (EEG) in normal rapid eye movement (REM) sleep. Black continuous arrows show some of the rapid eye movements in electrooculography and EEG; black dotted arrows highlight loss of electromyography (EMG) tone; **B,** EEG during REM behavior disorder. Black arrows show lack of atonia in EMG and increased EMG activity due to dream enacting behavior. EEG shows desynchronized normal pattern with no ictal epileptic rhythm. *(For color version, see Plate 4)*

(EMG) and electro-oculogram (EOG) recording, identification of REM sleep (Fig. 6a) and no loss of EMG tone in REM sleep will be obvious in REM parasomnia (Fig. 6b).

Confusional arousal is a form of NREM parasomnia seen in adulthood. This is due to brief and sudden awakening and this sudden state change leads onto brief confusion afterwards. From the history and witness account, it is difficult to differentiate from brief epileptic seizure with postictal confusion. Video EEG will be very useful to differentiate these two disorders clearly. Night terror is exclusively seen in children and not to be confused in adult patients.

In psychogenic nonepileptic attack disorders (NEAD), the video EEG show no ictal or postictal features of epileptic seizures. On many occasions, even though the history and eye witness account favors attacks arising from sleep, video EEG proves that the patient is awake with eyes closed at the onset of clinical attacks

(attacks from pseudo-sleep state) because of presence of awake EEG background such as posterior dominant alpha rhythm and absence of slow wave EEG features. Presence of α-rhythm thro' the muscle and movement artefacts during the attacks despite patient is unresponsive clinically also favors psychogenic nonepileptic attacks in sleep.

Excessive Daytime Sleepiness in People with Epilepsy

Excessive daytime sleepiness is commonly seen in people with epilepsy.[12] Both patients with focal epilepsy and generalized epilepsy have this morbidity. To some extent this is to do with seizure frequency, particularly nocturnal seizure frequency with disturbed night sleep. Apart from the common reasons for EDS in general population such as primary sleep disorders (OSA, PLMD, narcolepsy, circadian rhythm disturbances, and poor sleep hygiene), in the patients with epilepsy one need to consider other causes which include the role of anxiety or depression in the patients, type of antiepileptic medications (AEDs) and the number of AEDs, AED dose, seizure burden at night and also the role of epilepsy itself.

Epworth Sleepiness Scale (ESS) is a good clinical tool to assess EDS.[13] This questionnaire has eight components and each one has a score of 0–3 and total score possible is 24. A score of 0–9 is considered as normal. A score of 10 and above raises the suspicion of EDS and warrants investigation. Malow et al., using ESS found EDS is present in 28% of patients with epilepsy, whereas this is present only in 18% of patients with other neurological disorders.[14] Chen et al., calculated a prevalence of EDS in patients with epilepsy of 20%, whereas the prevalence in normal people is only 7%.[15] Hence, EDS is a significant comorbidity in people with epilepsy.

Factors to Consider if EDS is Present in a Person with Epilepsy

- Antiepileptic medications
- Comorbid psychiatric illness (anxiety and depressive illness)
- Nocturnal seizure burden and sleep disruption
- Coexistence of primary sleep disorders such as OSA, PLMD, narcolepsy, etc.
- Role of epilepsy itself.

Role of Antiepileptic Medications

All AEDs cause increase in fatigue and in higher dose cause excessive sleepiness. Those which cause increase in weight gain (phenobarbitone, levetiracetam, gabapentin, pregabalin, and perampanel) will aggravate OSA and contributes to EDS.[16] Benzodiazepines also worsens OSA but do not cause excessive weight gain. The other AEDs which can cause EDS are carbamazepine, oxcarbazepine, lacosamide, and zonisamide. These do not affect OSA. Lamotrigine can worsen insomnia. The effect of phenytoin and sodium valproate is variable on sleep. Felbamate is known to increase insomnia.

AED withdrawal also can affect sleep and opposite effects to the above mentioned are expected. Withdrawal of mood stabilizing AEDs such as valproate and lamotrigine can lead on to worsening anxiety or depression and this will affect the sleep pattern in the patients.

Circadian rhythm affects the AED absorption and metabolism. Generally, the serum levels are more with the same dose in the late evenings around 8 PM and this fact needs to be considered while AED prescription.[17]

Primary Sleep Disorders in People with Epilepsy (Fig. 7)

Primary sleep disorder such as OSA can co-exist with epilepsy and contribute to or can be the sole cause of EDS in patients with epilepsy[18] NREM and REM parasomnias can also co-exist with epilepsy. Nonrapid eye movement arousal disorders are common in people with NFLE. It may be impossible to diagnose or differentiate seizures disrupting the sleep and primary sleep disorders as a cause of patient's EDS and overnight PSG is needed in these cases (Fig. 7). Correct and prompt identification of primary sleep disorders in epilepsy is essential to treat

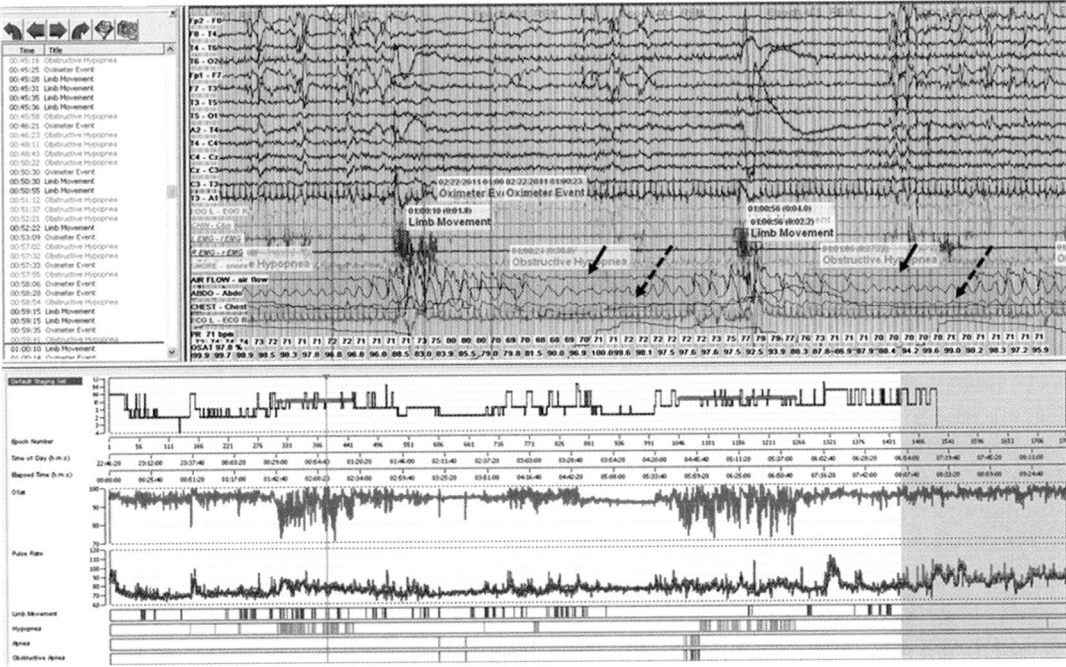

FIG. 7: An example slide for overnight polysomnography with hypnogram. Black arrows show absence of nasal airflow and dotted arrows show continuing chest and abdominal movements. This is typical pattern for obstructive sleep apnea. In central apnea, both airflow and chest/abdominal movements will be flat and unreactive during the periods of apnea. *(For color version, see Plate 5)*

effectively so that there will be improvement in both seizure control and QoL of these patients.

Berlin questionnaire[19] and STOP-BANG questionnaire[20] are good clinical tools for early diagnosis of OSA. A positive score in two out of three categories in Berlin questionnaire and an answer of YES to at least five out of eight questions in the updated STOP-BANG questionnaire raise the possibility of OSA and trigger investigation to confirm the diagnosis.

Manni et al. studied 283 adult patients with epilepsy and found 10.2% of these patients have OSA diagnosed by PSG studies.[21] Kaleyias et al. found 20% of children with epilepsy have coexistent OSA.[22] Primary sleep disorders need to be suspected in patients with epilepsy having EDS and particularly in those who have good seizure control, low AED dose or on monotherapy. Multiple sleep latency test (MSLT) is a good investigatory tool for the diagnosis of EDS.[23] The MSLT has five naps and a mean sleep onset latency of 5 minutes or less is pathological and supports EDS, particularly in those patients who had a total sleep time of >6 hours the previous night. Sleep onset REM (SOREM) is defined as occurrence of REM sleep within 15 minutes of sleep onset in an MSLT nap. Two or more SOREM in MSLT assessment along with pathologically short mean sleep onset latency are diagnostic of narcolepsy.

Occurrence of narcolepsy and epilepsy in a same patient has been reported in the literature. Periodic limb movement disorder and restless legs syndrome (RLS) are also can co-exist with epilepsy and will contribute to EDS if associated with increased arousal index in the PSG. Zonisamide, phenytoin, and ethosuximide can aggravate RLS. Antidepressants used to treat psychiatric comorbidities in sleep cause increase in RLS and PLMD in NREM sleep.

Treatment of sleep disorders improve seizure outcome and also QoL. Management of

OSA with continuous positive airway pressure (CPAP) has shown in improvements in seizure control with more AED responders.

The Effects of Epilepsy on Sleep Electroencephalography

Interictal epileptiform discharges are more common in N3 sleep and clinical seizures are more common in lighter (N1 and N2 sleep) stages of SWS or around the times where there is a state change between awake and sleep as well as from sleep to awake state. Seizures disrupt the sleep stages and architecture in the overnight sleep. Polysomnography studies have shown reduced REM sleep and increase in NREM sleep due to nocturnal seizures.[24] As REM sleep is vital for memory consolidation, memory impairment is common in people with epilepsy particularly with nocturnal seizures. Stereo EEG studies recently showed that in hippocampus increased synchronization of EEG rhythms occur even though the predominant finding in scalp EEG shows desynchronization.[25] This increased hippocampal synchronization supports memory consolidation in REM sleep. Seizures also lead on to reduced total sleep time, increased arousal index, poor sleep efficiency, and altered sleep architecture. The amount of N3 sleep (deeper stages of SWS) is less with epilepsy. This may explain the fatigue seen in people with epilepsy. Focal epilepsies particularly temporal lobe epilepsies disrupt sleep architecture more than frontal lobe seizures even though frontal lobe seizures are more frequently seen exclusively in sleep.

Role of Vagal Nerve Stimulation and Deep Brain Stimulation in Sleep

Medically intractable patients with epilepsy will be treated with vagal nerve stimulation (VNS) or deep brain stimulation (DBS of anterior nucleus of thalamus) with a view to reduce their seizure burden. Vagal nerve stimulation therapy increases SWS and reduces the number of arousals in the night sleep. These are partly related to improvement in seizure control. Unfortunately, VNS can reduce the airflow and increase the Apnea Hypopnea Index. In about 31% of patients treated with VNS, worsening of OSA or development of OSA may occur.[26] Hence, these patients need to be monitored for worsening of snoring or emergence of EDS. Ideally, PSG studies are needed prior to and after 3 months of VNS implantation to study the effect of VNS on breathing at least in patients with clinical suspicion. If needed, the stimulus frequency or the stimulation off time should be adjusted for the optimum effect without any side effects.

Deep brain stimulation of anterior nucleus of thalamus can increase the arousal level and hence increase the arousal index in the PSG. This may decrease the total sleep time and decrease the sleep efficiency.

Even though resective surgery is regularly performed in suitable refractory focal epilepsy patients, not much studies done to look into its role in sleep modification. Larger studies pre and postepilepsy surgery are needed to address this important aspect in patient management.

Practice Pearls in Recognizing and Treating Sleep Disorders in People with Epilepsy

- Watchful surveillance for EDS, worsening OSA, emergence of new type of nocturnal events
- Frontal lobe epilepsy and parasomnia scale, ESS questionnaire, and Berlin questionnaire, and STOP-BANG questionnaire
- Watchful eye particularly when there is AED change, AED withdrawal, VNS, and DBS treatments
- Monitoring weight gain change in mood
- Choosing less sedative AED (most newer AEDs), using extended release preparations, largest dose being at evenings and if possible monotherapy
- Encourage and reinforce sleep hygiene
  - No daytime naps
  - Regular sleep routine, optimum sleep environment
  - Avoid caffeinated drinks and large meals after 1800 hours.

CONCLUSION

The interaction between epilepsy and sleep are multifactorial, complex, and bidirectional. Optimal treatment for both disorders are important to effective patient management and to improve QoL. The above practice pearls will help in early recognition for the prompt management. Avoiding polypharmacy and choosing less central nervous system sedative AED medications and promoting sleep hygiene and regular sleep routines are all paramount for the patient management.

REFERENCES

1. Aristotle. On sleep and sleeplessness. [Beare JI, Trans.; 350 BCE] [cited 2018 Aug 11]. Available at: http://classics.mit.edu/Aristotle/sleep.html
2. Gowers WR. Epilepsy and other chronic convulsive diseases. New York: William Wood & Company; 1885. P. 162-4.
3. Langdon-Down M, Brain WR. Time of day in relation to convulsion in epilepsy. Lancet 1929;1:1029-32.
4. Gibbs EL, Gibbs FA. Diagnostic and localizing value of electroencephalographic studies in sleep. Res Publ Assoc Res Nerv Ment Dis. 1947;26:366-76.
5. Dennis GJ. The relationship between sleep and epilepsy. ACNR. 2016;16(2):13-6.
6. de Weerd A, de Haas S, Otte A, et al. Subjective sleep disturbance in patients with partial epilepsy: A questionnaire-based study on prevalence and impact on quality of life. Epilepsia. 2004;45(11):1397-404.
7. Kellaway P, Frost JD Jr, Crawley JW. Time modulation of ictal and interictal spike-and-wave activity in generalized epilepsy. Trans Am Neurol Assoc. 1979;104:92-3.
8. Shouse MN. Sleep deprivation increases susceptibility to kindled and penicillin seizure events during all waking and sleep states in cats. Sleep. 1988;11(2):162-71.
9. Kawahara R, Hamazaki Y, Takeshita H. Effect of REM sleep deprivation on the each seizure stage in feline amygdaloid kindling. Seishin Shinkeigaku Zasshi 1994;96(2):109-21.
10. Kreuzer P, Langguth B, Popp R, et al. Reduced intra-cortical inhibition after sleep deprivation: A transcranial magnetic stimulation study. Neurosci Lett. 2011;493(3):63-6.
11. Derry CP, Duncan JS, Berkovic SF. Paroxysmal motor disorders of sleep: The clinical spectrum and differentiation from epilepsy. Epilepsia. 2006;47(11):1775-91.
12. Sudha ST, Jeremy DS. Sleep and epilepsy. Sleep Med Clin. 2012(7);619-30.
13. Johns MW. A new method for measuring daytime sleepiness: The Epworth Sleepiness Scale. Sleep. 1991;14:50-5.
14. Malow BA, Bowes RJ, Lin X. Predictors of sleepiness in epilepsy patients. Sleep. 1997;20(12):1105-10.
15. Chen NC, Tsai MH, Chang CC, et al. Sleep quality and daytime sleepiness in patients with epilepsy. Acta Neurol Taiwan. 2011;20(4):249-56.
16. Jain SV, Glauser TA. Effects of epilepsy treatments on sleep architecture and daytime sleepiness: An evidence-based review of objective sleep metrics. Epilepsia. 2014;55(1):26-37.
17. Yegnanarayan R, Mahesh SD, Sangle S. Chronotherapeutic dose schedule of phenytoin and carbamazepine in epileptic patients. Chronobiol Int. 2006;23(5):1035-46.
18. Wyler AR, Weymuller EA Jr. Epilepsy complicated by sleep apnea. Ann Neurol. 1981;9(4):403-4.
19. Giorelli AS, Neves GS, Venturi M, et al. Excessive daytime sleepiness in patients with epilepsy: A subjective evaluation. Epilepsy Behav. 2011;21(4):449-52.
20. Chung F, Yang Y, Brown R, et al. Alternative scoring models of STOP-Bang questionnaire improve specificity to detect undiagnosed obstructive sleep apnea. J Clin Sleep Med. 2014;10(9):951-8.
21. Manni R, Politini L, Sartori I, et al. Daytime sleepiness in epilepsy patients: Evaluation by means of the Epworth Sleepiness Scale. J Neurol. 2000;247(9):716-7.
22. Kaleyias J, Cruz M, Goraya JS. Spectrum of polysomnographic abnormalities in children with epilepsy. Pediatr Neurol. 2008;39(3):170-6.
23. Littner MR, Kushida C, Wise M, et al. Practice parameters for clinical use of the multiple sleep latency test and the maintenance of wakefulness test. Sleep. 2005;28(1):113-21.
24. Bazil CW, Castro LH, Walczak TS. Reduction of rapid eye movement sleep by diurnal and nocturnal seizures in temporal lobe epilepsy. Arch Neurol. 2000;57(3):363-8.
25. Moroni F, Nobili L, Curcio G, et al. Sleep in the human hippocampus: A stereo-EEG study. PLoS ONE. 20017;2(9):e867.
26. Marzec M, Edwards J, Sagher O, et al. Effects of vagus nerve stimulation on sleep-related breathing in epilepsy patients. Epilepsia. 2003;44(7):930-5.

CHAPTER 4

Granulomas of Nontuberculous and Noncystisercal Origin

Suresh C Thirunavukarasu, Paranjothi Shanmugam

INTRODUCTION

Mononuclear predominant inflammatory cells occurring focally is defined as a granuloma. Granuloma is a protective mechanism in which the inflammatory response is unable to destroy the invading antigen which could be an infectious organism, chemical agent, antigen, or a foreign body.[1]

After initial infection, the macrophages migrate to the infection site from the blood. They have various innate immune receptors in their membranes, allowing them to recognize bacteria, take them up by phagocytosis, and secrete various cytokines. The complex interaction between activated macrophages, T lymphocytes mediated by a variety of cytokines results in T lymphocyte proliferation and activation at sites of antigen deposition. The T-cell induces interleukin-1 on the macrophage and thereafter a cavalcade of chemotactic factors promotes granulomagenesis. Interferon-γ increases the expression of MHC class II molecules on macrophages, and activated macrophage receptors carry an Fc fraction of IgG to potentiate their ability to phagocytose. The end product is the granuloma.

Infectious diseases, vasculitis, immunological mechanisms, leucocyte oxidase defect, hypersensitivity, chemicals, and malignancies can incite T-cell mediated response and cause granuloma formation.

Four groups of granulomas are identified and they are granulomas secondary to T-cell mediated response to an infectious agent.

Granulomas with a T-cell mediated response but where the cause is not known.

A foreign body response culminates in the formation of granuloma.

Lastly tumors also can end up forming granulomas. This classification is slightly modified from the previous classification in which three groups were propounded. Group 1: granulomas are secondary to a specific organism. Group 2 is secondary to an organism which is diagnosed by molecular diagnostic methods and group 3 is in which an etiology is suspected but not proved by available diagnostic methods.[2]

Though tuberculous granulomas are commonly encountered nontuberculous and non cystisercous granulomas are not infrequent and causes significant morbidity and if untreated mortality. It consists of only 5% of total granulomas and diagnosis of this subgroup remains a challenge.[3] In this review article we will try to discuss in brief the etiopathogenesis, clinical features, and treatment aspects of nontuberculous and noncystisercous granulomas of infectious and immunological origin.

GRANULOMAS OF BRAIN SECONDARY TO INFECTIONS

Bacterial Infections

Neuroborreliosis

In the United States, 200,000 cases of Lyme disease have been reported to the Centers for Disease Control, resulting in a national incidence of 9.7 cases per 100 000 population. It's a tick borne disease transmitted by the bite of Ixodes ticks.

Clinical Features

In the United States, erythema migrans rash, arthritis, and carditis are common presentations. In Europe and Asia, radiculitis and acrodermatitis chronica atrophicans are more common presenting signs.

In India Lyme disease cases have been reported in Kerala and Haryana.[4,5]

The pathogenesis and clinical symptoms are different between American and European patients. In Europe the central nervous system (CNS) spread is via the nerves and hence the common clinical presentation is radicular pain and myelitis which is called as Bannwarth syndrome.[5]

In American patients it is blood spread and the clinical presentation is mild confusion to severe encephalitis.

The spectrum of neurological manifestations could be cerebral involvement manifesting as drowsiness to encephalitis, spinal cord involvement causing transverse myelitis. Peripheral nervous system (PNS) involvement results in painful radiculopathy, ocular, and orbital involvement causing optic neurpathy, uveitis, conjunctivitis, and orbital myositis.

Headache is the most frequent neurologic symptom in the pediatric population. The most common neurologic signs of pediatric neuroborreliosis include facial nerve palsy (3–5%) and meningitis (1%). Less common manifestations are sleep disturbance and papilledema associated with increased intracranial pressure. Ataxia, chorea, myelitis, pseudotumor cerebri, meningitis, and encephalopathy are very uncommon.

A subgroup of patients may present with cognitive and neuropsychiatric disturbance which falls into the spectrum of "chronic neuroborreliosis".

Fatigue, paresthesias, difficulty in sleeping, cognitive impairment, headache, arthralgia and myalgia persist for more than 6 months after standard treatment of neuro Lyme disease or other clearly defined Lyme disease manifestations, the condition is often termed post-Lyme disease syndrome.[7]

Diagnosis

Magnetic resonance imaging (MRI) may show lesions similar to multiple sclerosis including involvement of calloso septal interface but periventicular involvement is uncommon in Lyme disease.[6]

Detection of antibodies against Lyme disease by a two-step test involving enzyme immuneassay and enzyme-linked immunosorbent assay (ELISA) and a final confirmation by Western blot is routinely used.

Recent studies have suggested that the B-cell attracting chemokine CXCL13 which is increased in the cerebrospinal fluid (CSF) of patients with early neuroborreliosis.

The following three criteria should be present for definite neuroborreliosis: (i) neurological symptoms; (ii) CSF pleocytosis; (iii) Borrelia-specific antibodies produced intrathecally.[6]

Treatment

Early neuroborreliosis with manifestations confined to the PNS and meninges:

Oral doxycycline or intravenous ceftriaxone or intravenous penicillin or intravenous cefotaxime are effective and safe treatments.

Oral doxycycline (200 mg daily) and intravenous ceftriaxone (2 g daily) for 14 days are equally effective. The advantages of doxycycline are the oral route of administration and the lower costs. Doxycycline is relatively contraindicated during pregnancy or lactation.

Early neuroborreliosis with CNS symptoms, intravenous ceftriaxone for 3 weeks though some tend to manage the same way as neuroborreliosis confined to PNS and meninges.

Adult patients with definite or possible late neuroborreliosis with peripheral neuropathy should be treated with oral doxycycline (200 mg daily) or intravenous ceftriaxone (2 g daily) for 3 weeks.

Adult patients with definite or possible late LNB with CNS manifestations (myelitis, encephalitis, vasculitis) should be treated with intravenous ceftriaxone (2 g daily) for 3 weeks.[7]

Key points

- Uncommon in India neuroborreliosis has different spectrum of pathogenesis and clinical manifestations in European and American patients
- Apart from neuropathy, meningitis, and myelitis a sub group of patients may have late neuroborreliosis which manifests with neuropsychiatric manifestations
- Post-Lyme disease syndrome can occur 6 months after corrective treatment
- MRI often mimics MS lesions but absence of periventricular involvement aids the diagnosis
- Antibodies against borrelia and CXCL13 detection is useful in detecting early Lyme diseases
- Treatment is with doxycycline and ceftriaxone which is tailored according to early and late neuroborreliosis

Neurobrucellosis

Brucellosis is a zoonotic illness which gains access to human being after intake of contaminated or unpasteurized milk.

It primarily involves the reticuloendothelial system and affects other systems as well.

Neurological complications are noted in 0–25% of patients, more common in adults, and in male population.[8]

Clinical Features

Headache, seizures, meningitis, meningoencephalitis, basal meningitis causing cranial nerve palsies are frequent presentations.

Arterial and venous strokes have also been reported with neurobrucellosis.

Involvement of spinal cord may result in transverse myelitis and spinal arachnoiditis.

Diagnosis

Diagnosis is established by a diagnostic criteria which includes the following:
- Signs and symptoms of neurological disease in the absence of other diseases
- Isolation of bacteria from blood and other body fluids
- Standard tube agglutination titers positivity in serum and/or cerebrospinal fluid
- Cerebrospinal fluid shows evidence of chronic meningitis with raised lymphocytes and protein and decreased glucose levels.

Presence of any one of the above mentioned criteria is sufficient for diagnosing brucellosis.

However, diagnosis is frequently established by the clinical features, serum agglutinin titer of >1:160 in tube agglutination titer and a positive blood culture.

Magnetic resonance imaging may show normal findings, evidence of meningeal enhancement due to chronic meningitis, white matter changes mimicking demyelination and vascular changes which could be confined to arterial or venous territory.

Treatment

Treatment of neurobrucellosis usually involves dual or triple combination of antibiotics. Doxycycline, rifampicin, trimethoprim-sulfamethoxazole, streptomycin, or ceftriaxone is used for more than 2 months.

However, the exact combination of antibiotics and the required duration of treatment are controversial. However, the duration is more than 8 weeks and in some studies it can be given up to 6 months. If ceftriaxone injections are used in treatment the duration of treatment may be shortened.

Key points

- Neuroborreliosis occurs between 0 and 25% of patients with borreliosis
- Central nervous system involvement includes meningitis, headache, seizures, myelopathy, and cranial nerve palsies
- A consistent diagnostic criterion is available for the diagnosis

- Combination of antibiotics for more than 8 weeks which can go up to 6 months is commonly used
- The commonest combination of triple antibiotic therapy was doxycycline, rifampin, and cotrimoxazole

Neurosyphilis

Syphilis is a sexually transmitted disease caused by *Treponema pallidum*. Invasion of the CNS occurs early in the course of untreated syphilis. Neurosyphilis is defined as a CSF WBC count of 20 cells/µL or greater and a reactive CSF venereal disease research laboratory test result. *T. pallidum* gains access to the body by way of minute abrasions of the skin or mucous membranes. Attachment to host cells involves the action of a mucopolysaccharidase. The pathogenesis is primarily obliterative endarteritis of terminal arterioles with resultant inflammatory and necrotic changes. Syphilis is classified as primary, secondary, tertiary, or quaternary. Tertiary lesions are caused by obliterative small vessel endarteritis, which usually involves the vasa vasorum of the CNS. The US Centers for Disease Control and Prevention (CDC) criteria has classified neurosyphilis into 3 forms namely, neuropsychiatric, meningovascular and myelopathic.[9]

Neurosyphilis is divided into two general categories: (i) early involvement of the CNS limited to the meninges, and (ii) parenchymal involvement. It can be:

1. Asymptomatic
2. Acute syphilitic meningitis
3. Meningovascular syphilis
4. Tabes dorsalis
5. General paresis
6. Optic atrophy.

- *Asymptomatic neurosyphilis:* Asymptomatic neurosyphilis is characterized by a reactive nontreponemal CSF serology (VDRL test) without clinical manifestations
- *Acute syphilitic meningitis:* Patients with acute syphilitic meningitis have signs of meningeal irritation, stiff neck, headache, nausea, and vomiting with cranial nerve involvement. Fever is conspicuously absent
- *Meningovascular syphilis:* Endarteritis and luminal narrowing causes ischemic strokes. Middle cerebral artery (MCA) and basilar artery are commonly involved. Meningeal neurosyphilis usually manifests with clinical features of acute meningitis, including hydrocephalus, cranial neuropathies, seizures, and the formation of leptomeningeal granulomas, called gummas. A gumma is a well-circumscribed mass of avascular granulation tissue. It results from a cell-mediated immune response to *T. pallidum*. Gummas usually are extra-axial lesions and are dura based. The cortex is often involved secondary to local extension and mass effect[10]
- *Tabes dorsalis*: Tabes dorsalis is a slowly progressive parenchymatous degenerative disease involving the posterior columns and posterior roots of the spinal cord. Patients usually present with loss of pain sensation, loss of peripheral reflexes, rhombergism, and progressive ataxia. Bladder incontinence and loss of sexual function are common. The 3 stages of tabes dorsalis are preataxia, ataxia, and paralysis. The characteristic gait is wide-based and high stamping. Charcot joints and trophic ulcers often develop due to proprioceptive loss [11-13]
- *General Paresis of the insane*: Cognitive dysfunction with memory disturbance, irritability, and depression is due to chronic progressive frontotemporal meningoencephalitis. Pathologically, this type is characterized by a perivascular and meningeal chronic inflammatory reaction with meningeal fibrosis, granular ependymitis, degeneration of the cortical parenchyma and tissue invasion with spirochetes
- *Optic atrophy*: Panuveitis and optic neuropathy could be granulomatous, retinitis and papillitis.

Diagnosis

Serological testing, dark-field microscopy of the skin lesions, and biopsy with direct fluorescent antibody staining of material from the lesion is used in the diagnosis of syphilis. The fluorescent trepenomal antibody absorption test and the MHA-TP are reactive and helps in confirmation of the disease.[14]

Cerebrospinal Fluid Findings

The diagnosis of neurosyphilis is based on a CSF WBC count of 20 cells/μL or greater, and/or a reactive CSF VDRL, and/or a positive CSF intrathecal *T. pallidum* antibody index.[14]

Imaging Studies

MRI brain shows fronto cortical atrophy, T2 hyperintensity could be patchy or diffuse, mesiotemporal T2 hyperintensity, dilated ventricles, and pathological T2 hypointensity of the globus pallidus, putamen, head of the caudate, and thalamus. Cerebral syphilitic gumma, shows juxtacortical location with nodular enhancement and shows moderately restriction on diffusion. Dural tail and surrounding vasogenic edema are characteristic for dural based location of Gumma. They densely enhance with contrast. Single-photon emission computed tomography (SPECT) is a useful method for evaluating an inflammatory state and for assessing the effect of therapy on neurosyphilis. Increased cerebral blood flow is detected by iodine-123 N-isopropyl-p-iodoamphetamine SPECT, consistent with the active inflammatory state of neurosyphilis. On successful treatment the increased blood flow is decreased.[11-13]

Magnetic resonance imaging in syphilitic myelitis demonstrates high-intensity areas on T2-weighted images similar to transverse myelitis.

In meningovascular syphilis, MRI shows meningeal enhancement and T2 hyperintensity with diffusion restriction in the arterial artery. CT scan shows hypodense areas suggestive of ischemic infarction in vascular territories. Magnetic resonance angiography has demonstrated irregularities of the involved artery suggesting arteritis.

Treatment

Aqueous crystalline penicillin G 18–24 million units per day, given as continuous infusion or given as 3–4 million units every 4 hours.

If compliance can be ensured, procaine penicillin G 2.4 million units intramuscularly once daily along with probenecid 500 mg four times a day.

Both the regimens are continued for 2 weeks.

All persons should be tested for human immunodeficiency virus (HIV) status. If CSF had shown pleocytosis before treatment repeat CSF examination is done after 6 months to ensure cell count becomes normal and nontrepenomal CSF VDRL titers decreases four fold.[14]

Persons with HIV infection and neurosyphilis should be treated according to the recommendations for HIV-negative persons with neurosyphilis.

In patients who have allergy to penicillin ceftriaxone 2 g daily either intramuscular or intravenous for 10–14 days can be used as an alternative treatment for persons with neurosyphilis.

> **Key points**
> - Central nervous system involvement occurs early in the disease
> - Neurological and radiological manifestations are protean involving meninges, arteries, parenchyma, cranial nerves and spinal cord
> - Diagnosis is achieved using treponemal and nontreponemal tests
> - Longer duration of treatment with penicillin to the extent of two weeks is required for neurosyphilis and in patients allergic to penicillin, ceftrioxone is used

Actinomycosis

Actinomycosis is a noncontagious, slow suppurative bacterial infection caused by *Actinomyces israelii*. These organisms are classified as gram-positive, non-acid fast branching filamentous bacteria with anaerobic or microaerophilic requirements.

The primary focus of infection is lungs or liver from which brain is infected by hemotogenous spread. Contiguous spread via sinuses and bones also occur.

Clinical Features

It could be meningitic and nonmeningitic forms.

The meningitic form presents with classical features of chronic fever and signs of meningeal irritation while the non meningitic form presents with brain abcess, space occupying lesions, subdural empyema, and an epidural abcess. Cerebral abscesses are usually singular, multiloculated, encapsulated and unencapsulated. There is a predilection for involvement of the temporal and frontal lobes.[15,16]

Diagnosis

Magnetic resonance imaging is an important mode of investigation though it may not be of value in telling the etiology of the abscess. Diffusion restriction and low apparent diffusion coefficient (ADC) levels and high ADC with no restriction within the abscess cavity and wall of the abscess are the characteristic findings in MRI. The reverse happens in malignancies.[17]

Elevated aminoacids, acetate, and succinate may give a clue for the actinomycotic abscess.

Biopsy showing gram positive filamentous rods gives the confirmatory diagnosis.

Treatment

High dose penicillin therapy along with surgical debridement is the preferred treatment.

Intravenous penicillin G 24 million units/day for 8 weeks.

It is followed by an oral dose of amoxicillin for 4 months.

For abscesses surgical debridement is done in selected cases.

> **Key points**
> - Central nervous system actinomycosis take up meningeal and nonmeningeal forms
> - Invasion of central nervous system is via blood or by contiguous spread
> - Abscesses do occur and has a predilection for temporal and frontal lobes
> - Magnetic resonance imaging and magnetic resonance spectroscopy are complimentary for the diagnosis and biopsy is the mainstay for diagnosis
> - High dose penicillin for 8 weeks followed by oral antibiotics for months along with surgical debridement if required is treatment of choice

Leprosy

Leprosy is a chronic infectious disease caused by *Mycobacterium leprae*, an acid-fast, rod-shaped bacillus. The disease mainly affects the skin, the peripheral nerves, mucosa of the upper respiratory tract, and the eyes.

India accounts for 58.85% of new cases in the world. In the year 2013–14, 1.27 lakh new cases were reported in India based on WHO statistics.

The accepted classification was propounded by Rudling and Jopling which is based on clinical, histological and immunological criteria.

Tuberculoid, borderline tuberculoid, borderline, borderline lepromatous, lepromatous, and indeterminate are different subgroups of patients classified based on the immunological state of the patient.

In lepromatous leprosy macrophages are unable to kill the bacilli while in bordeline patients there is an immune cell mediated response to destroy the bacteria.

A clinical presentation of leprosy without any skin lesions known as "pure neuritic form". There is also a condition known as "silent neuropathy". It is characterized by the impairment of sensory and motor functions without skin signs, nerve tenderness, pain, paresthesia or numbness symptoms of neuritis. It is also called "quiet nerve paralysis".[18]

Clinical Features

The common neurological manifestation is involvement of nerves which is usually sensory, followed by motor nerves. Spectrum of involvement could be mononeuropathy, mononeuritis multiplex, and symmetrical neuropathy. Ulnar and common peroneal nerves are commonly involved. Anesthetic hypopigmented patches, wasting, and weakness causing clawing and foot drop are common clinical manifestations.

Because of sensory impairment ulcers, trophic changes, and Charcot joints occur.

Type 1 as well as type 2 lepra reaction involves the peripheral nerves and it is characterised by pain, nerve involvement, and foot drop or clawing.

Great auricular nerve, supraclavicular nerve, ulnar nerves, dorsal cutaneous nerve of ulnar nerve, medial, and superficial radial nerves, femoral and common peroneal nerves, superficial peroneal nerve, posterior tibial nerves, and sural nerves are commonly enlarged.

Weakness and wasting are proportionate with degree of involvement of nerves.

Cranial nerve involvement occurs in 18% of leprosy patients. The fifth and seventh cranial nerves are the most affected. Isolated sixth cranial nerve involvement is secondary to type1 lepra reaction and a multiple cranial nerve palsy simulating Melkerson-Rosenthal syndrome is also reported in literature.

A subgroup of patients develop delayed nerve impairment years after multiple drug therapy, which could not be explained by relapses or reactions. They have acute mononeuropathy or slowly progressive form of multiple mononeuropathy or polyneuropathy. This subgroup is leprosy late-onset neuropathy in which there is no active leprosy.[19]

Small fiber neuropathy with pain and a case of complex regional pain syndrome secondary to Hansen's disease have been reported as well.

Diagnosis

Computerized quantitative sensory tests for small fibers, contact heat evoked potentials for somatosensory pathways and corneal confocal microscopy for unmyelinated fibers of cornea are new tools for aiding the diagnosis of leprosy.

Clinical features of hypopigmented patch, nerve thickening, and demonstration of acid fast bacilli in biopsied specimens are diagnostic of leprosy.

Treatment

Multibacillary leprosy (MB): For adults the standard regimen is rifampicin 600 mg once a month, dapsone 100 mg daily, clofazimine 300 mg once a month, and 50 mg daily. Duration is for 12 months.

Paucibacillary leprosy (PB): For adults the standard regimen is rifampicin 600 mg once a month, dapsone: 100 mg, daily duration is for 6 months.

Single skin lesion paucibacillary leprosy: For adults the standard regimen is a single dose of rifampicin 600 mg ofloxacin 400 mg minocycline 100 mg.

Minocycline and oflaxacin can be given in patients who do not tolerate clofazamine.

> **Key points**
> - Approximately 58% of cases are reported from India
> - Clinical subtypes are based on the immune status of the patient
> - Nerve involvement could be mononeuropathy, multiple neuropathies, small fiber neuropathy, and symmetrical neuropathy
> - Silent neuropathy and neuritic form are also noted clinical presentations of Hansen's disease
> - Diagnosis is clinical while electromyography and biopsy is done in selected cases and if required

Rhinoscleroma

Rhinoscleroma is a chronic granulomatous disease affecting the upper respiratory tract.

The disease is endemic in Egypt and it is prevelant in north India.[20] *Klebsiella rhinoscleromatis* also called as Frisch bacillus is the causative organism.

Clinical Features

The disease has three stages: (i) Catarrhal stage, characterized by purulent nasal discharge and crusting, (ii) granulomatous stage, in which painless and nonulcerative granulomatous nodules form in the nasal mucosa along with subdermal infiltration of the external nose and upper lip. A typical hebra nose could be the end result and (iii) cicatricial stage, causes stenosis of the nares, distortion of the face and lips with adhesions in the nose, nasopharynx, and oropharynx.

Invasion into the orbit and skull base is extremely rare and only three cases exist in literature with intracranial involvement. CNS involvement is by invading the brain via cribiform plate giving rise to tumor like masses, involving the cavernous sinus and left MCA causing infarction.

Diagnosis

Histopathology shows inflammatory cells, Russell bodies, and the characteristic Mickulicz cells. These cells are very characteristic of rhinoscleroma though not specific.[20]

Treatment

Treatment should include long-term antimicrobial therapy and surgical intervention in patients with symptoms of obstruction.

Long term antibiotics used are tetracycline, ciprofloxacin and third generation cephalosporins. Sclerotic lesions respond well to quinolones.

Bacterial over infection responds to treatment with third-generation cephalosporins and clindamycin.

Long-term antibiotic therapy often eradicates this infection. Surgical management is by a team comprising neuro, ENT and plastic surgeons and tailored according to patient's requirement.

Key points

- Only few case reports of neurological involvement secondary to rhinoscleroma has been reported
- Histopathology demonstrating Mickulicz cells is characteristic of this disease
- Treatment is by combination of long term medical treatment with surgical intervention

Cat Scratch Disease

First described in 1950, cat scratch disease, is caused by an organism *Bartonella henselae*.

Exposure to cat by way of its scratch or bite can cause cat scratch disease. Cat flea or ticks also can cause this self-limiting disease which usually causes a regional lymphadenitis.

Neuropathogeneis is not clear but *B. henselae* can attack and colonize dendritic cells, CD34 progenitor cells, erythrocytes and vascular endothelial cells, triggering cell mediated immunity and granuloma formation.

Clinical Features

Neurological involvement occurs only in 2% of patients.

Encephalopathy is the commonest presentation followed by seizures, myelitis, radiculopathy, radiculomyeloencephalopathy, and cranial nerve palsies.[21,22]

Neuroretinits and a case of chronic demyelinating neuropathy have been reported secondary to cat scratch disease.

Diagnosis

Cerebrospinal fluid, electroencephalograph and neuroimaging are nonspecific. Bacterial isolation, polymerase chain amplification and cloning may supplant the clinical criteria used in diagnosing cat scratch disease.

Three of the following four criteria should be met and they are:
1. Contact with a cat and presence of a scratch or primary lesion
2. Exclusion of other causes of lymphadenopathy
3. A positive skin test
4. A characteristic histopathology.

Treatment

Treatment includes antibiotics which doxycycline, azithromycin, rifampicin, levofloxacin alone or in combinations for more than 6 weeks. Steroids for myelitis and neuroretinitis can be used.

Plasmapheresis if necessary and anticonvulsants for seizures are given.

Key points

- Neurological manifestations occur only in 2% of patients with cat scratch disease
- Encephalopathy and neuroretinitis are common clinical presentations
- Azithromycin and doxycycline either alone or in combinations are used in treatment

Parasitic Infections

Schistosomiasis

Blood flukes are *Schistosoma mansoni, japonicum* and *haemotobium*. They access CNS when eggs of the worms are laid ectopically.

Eggs reach CNS either by retrograde flow or by the worms themselves when they reach hemotogenously.

This can cause, myelitis, radiculopathy, arteritis, and granulomatous reaction in the involved areas.

Clinical Features

Myelopathy and radiculopathy occur together and the classical presentation is cauda conus presentation. It is characterized by root pain, weakness, bladder, and bowel involvement. The granulomatous form also can cause intra axial and extra axial lesions.

Cerebral schistosomiasis usually presents as a space occupying lesion and it is very rare. It is seen in only 2-4 % of *Schistosoma japonicum* patients. Clinical manifestations are seizures, headache, features of raised intracranial hypertension, and weakness.[23]

Computed tomography and MRI will aid in the diagnosis and not specific.

Magnetic resonance imaging shows medullary cone enlargement and when this MRI feature is seen in an endemic area of schistosomiasis needle of suspicion on medullary schistosomiasis becomes high.

A linear pattern surrounded by tree like punctiform pattern is highly suggestive if not specific for schistosomiasis. Multiple intensely enhancing nodules in clusters similar to "Buddha's hand" appearance or arborizing pattern, is located in the cerebral white matter and basal ganglia. This MRI pattern is shown in Fig. 1 and is highly suggestive of cerebral schistosomiasis.[24]

Treatment

Praziquantel along with steroids and in selected cases neurosurgical intervention is the treatment option for cerebral schistosomiasis.

> **Key points**
> - Around 2–4 % of patients with schistosomiasis develop neurological manifestation
> - Common clinical presentations are cauda conus presentation and seizures
> - Medullary cone enlargement in an endemic area and "Buddha's hand" appearance in cerebral white matter are important clues in MRI to diagnose cerebral schistosomiasis
> - Praziquantel is the drug of choice for schistosomiasis

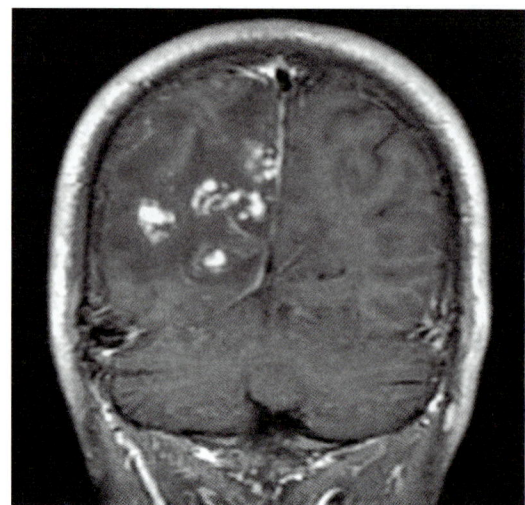

FIG. 1: Multiple nodular enhancing lesions–Buddha's hand appearance.

Cerebral Paragonimasis

Cerebral paragonimasis has been described as the most common and serious form of extrapulmonary paragonimasis, which is common in China and Japan. In India, north eastern states like Manipur and Nagaland have high incidence of paraganimasis.[30]

The encysted metacercaria found in the poorly cooked crab and crayfish infests the mammalian host. The larva usually penetrates the diaphragm and gets access to lungs.

The cerebral infection has been described due to erratic migration of the worms which enter the cranial cavity through the jugular or carotid foramen and then invades the temporal and occipital lobes.

Clinical Features

Clinical features are nonspecific and may present with headache, seizures, and focal neurological deficits.

Diagnosis

The most common imaging findings of cerebral paragonimiasis are isodense or hypodense lesions combined with extensive hypodense areas of perilesional edema on CT scans and a large mass composed of multiple ring-shaped lesions with surrounding edema on MRI images. The conglomeration of multiple ring-shaped lesions giving rise to "soap bubble appearance". "Tunnel signs" (Fig. 2) due to the tracking of the worm and "worm-eaten sign" were characteristic of most CP images.[26]

In India, Regional Medical Research Centre, Dibrugarh has developed IgG ELISA using E/S antigen for diagnosis of paragonimiasis. It is highly sensitive and specific.

Treatment

Praziquantel at 25 mg/kg body weight administered orally three times a day after meals for three days without any appreciable side effects. With this regimen relapse occurred in about 2% cases. A 100% cure rate was obtained when the therapy was extended up to 5 days.

Praziquantel has replaced the older drug bithional which had urticaria as a common side effect.

Key points

- Paragonimus infection is more common in China and Japan and in India, north eastern states have high incidence of this disease
- Central nervous system infection usually occurs in occipital and temporal lobes and MRI shows typical signs like soap bubble appearance and tunnel signs
- Praziquantel is the drug of choice and it is well tolerated and complete cure occurs when treatment is extended for 5 days

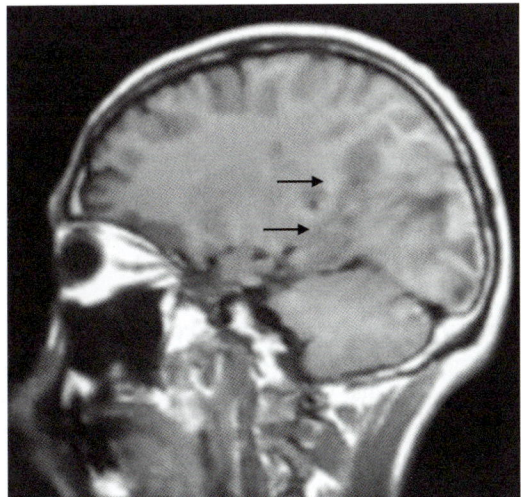

FIG. 2: Magnetic resonance imaging shows Tunnel sign which indicates the path traversed by the parasite.

Granulomatous Amebic Encephalitis

Free-living amoebae are *Acanthomeba* sp, *Balamuthia mandrillaris* and Sapinna pedata. They enter the CNS hemotogenously from lung, genitounrinary tract, and skin. Balamuthiasis infection is usually preceded by skin infection.

Clinical Features

The disease is usually chronic or subacute encephalitis and clinical presentation is lethargy, seizures, low grade fever, signs of raised intracranial pressure, and cerebrovascular accidents due to amebic arteritis.

In CNS infections, the most common affected regions are the cerebral hemispheres, thalamus, cerebellum, and midbrain. Lesions are usually necrotic and hemorrhagic granulomatous material are seen during resection.

Computed tomography scan and MRI may show multiple or single lesion with contrast enhancement and some may mimic an abscess.[27-29]

Cerebrospinal fluid may show mononuclear pleocytosis, raised protein and decreased glucose.

Demonstration of trophozoites in the lesion, skin, and lungs will give the definitive diagnosis.

Treatment is usually a combination of antibiotics, pentamidine, cotrimoxazole, propamidine isethionate, azoles like fluconazole, itraconazole, and voriconazole, amphotericin B, flucytosine and rifampin, azithromycin, amikacin.

Usually four antibiotics are combined. Along with this neurosurgical procedures are done in selected cases.

Despite this the survival in granulomatous amebic encephalitis is dismal.

Key points

- Granulomatous amebic encephalitis usually causes encephalitis and strokes due to arteritis
- Single or multiple lesions mimicking an abscess are seen in neuroimaging
- Demonstration of trophozoites gives the definitive diagnosis
- Combination of antibiotics is usually used in treating this often fatal disease

Echinococcosis

In India, the hydatid disease is commonly seen in the Kurnool district of Andhra Pradesh, Madurai district of Tamil Nadu and in Punjab.[30]

Echinococcus granulosus, alveolaris, and *multilocularis* are tapeworms which infests human beings when they eat food items which are contaminated by the eggs of tapeworm. The eggs release oncospheres in the intestine which gains access to portal circulation and reach liver and then lung. CNS involvement is rare, and it is roughly 1-2 %of patients with echinococcosis .They reach the brain via blood. Rupture of cysts and embolization also can reach the brain.

The cysts which are formed by direct seeding are called primary hydatid cyst, they are fertile and usually single.

The embolized cysts from elsewhere are infertile and may be multiple. They don't have scolices.

Clinical Features

Neurological manifestations primarily depends on the area involved and are headache, features of raised intracranial tension like vomiting and papilledema, focal neurological deficits.[30]

Spinal cord is involved and it is less than 1%. Thoracic followed by lumbar and sacral segments are usually involved and it causes cortical bony erosions.

Diagnosis

Magnetic resonance imaging as shown in fig. 3 gives valuable information in the diagnosis of cerebral hydatid with intraxial cystic lesion in the territory of middle cerebral artery (MCA), with minimal or no perilesional edema. The cyst fluid is isointense to CSF in all pulse sequences. MRS shows elevation of lactate, alanine, acetate, and pyruvate. Elevation of pyruvate is different from other cystic lesions.

Treatment

The treatment of hydatid cyst is surgical and the aim of surgery is to excise the cyst in toto without rupture, to prevent recurrence and anaphylactic reaction.

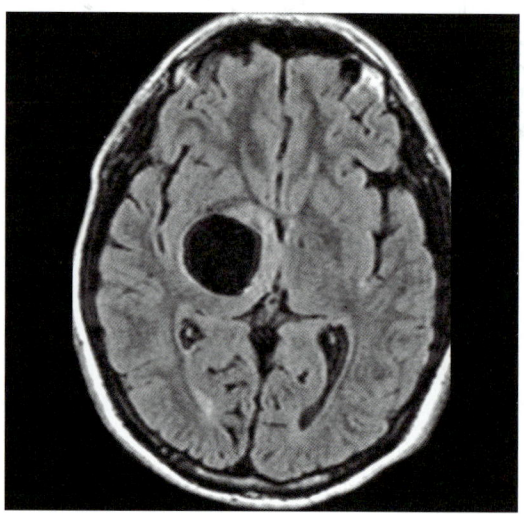

FIG. 3: The FLAIR magnetic resonance imaging showing the cyst with no perilesional edema. The cyst is isointense to cerebrospinal fluid in all sequences.

Albendazole at 10 mg/kg body weight thrice a day for four months showed disappearance of cysts in a few case reports.

Surgical and medical therapy can be combined together for better results in preventing recurrence.

Key points

- Hydatid cysts could be primary or secondary which accesses brain by blood or by embolization
- Central nervous system involvement occurs in 1–2%of patients and clinical manifestations occur pertaining to the area of involvement of the hydatid cyst
- Magnetic resonance imaging shows cysts which are isointense to cerebrospinal fluid and there is minimal perilesional edema
- The consensus treatment is albendazole along with complete excision of the cyst

Central Nervous System Toxoplasmosis

The CNS toxoplasmosis is more common in patients with HIV infection. In India it is between 1.33–3.33%. In Indian population CNS toxoplasmosis in immunocompetent person is very rare and worldwide it is 0.018%.

Definitive hosts are kitten and they excrete diploid cysts formed from gametocytes. Excreted sporulated cysts are infective and they become sporozoites in intestine .They penetrate in intestinal wall and enter tissues like skeletal muscle and remain dormant. When the immunity is compromised they multiply actively and are called tachyzoites. They invade CNS and have a predilection for basal ganglia, corticomedullary junction, white matter, and periventricular regions.

Clinical Features

Clinical manifestations of CNS toxoplasmosis include headache, seizures, cranial nerve palsies, and meningoencephalitis and focal deficits. Chorioretinitis and meningoencephalitis are common clinical presentations of CNS toxoplasmosis and after the advent of HIV infection the commonest cause of cerebral mass lesion in HIV patients is due to toxoplasmosis.[31,32]

Diagnosis

Multiple T2 hyperintense lesions with basal ganglia and periventricular predilection and ring enhancement in contrast weighted imaging gives a clue for CNS toxoplasmosis. Fig. 4 shows ring enhancement and periventricular involvement. On T1 weighted images presence of peripheral hyperintensity, due to hemorrhage helps to differentiate from CNS lymphoma which also has a propensity to involve periventricular regions. Lipid lactate peak in MRS also gives a clue for CNS toxoplasmosis.[32]

Treatment

In immunocompetent patients the six week regimen includes pyrimethamine 100 mg as loading dose followed by 25-50 mg/day along with pyrimethamine either sulfadiazine at 2-4 g/day or clindamycin 300 mg four times a day. Folinic acid 10-25 mg/day is added to the regimen to prevent pyrimethamine induced bone marrow suppression. Trimethoprim (10 mg/kg/day) along with sulfamethoxazole (50 mg/kg/day) for 4 weeks.

In pregnant women spiramycin 1 gm orally every 8 hours is given and in patients with AIDS pyrimethamine 200 mg initially followed by 50-75 mg/day along with sulfadiazine 4-8 g/day for 6 weeks followed by lifelong suppression or until immune reconstitution. If CD4 count is less than 100 suppressive therapy with pyrimethamine 50 mg/day plus sulfadiazine 1-1.5 g/day is given for life or until immune reconstitution. Folinic acid is routinely added to this regimen.

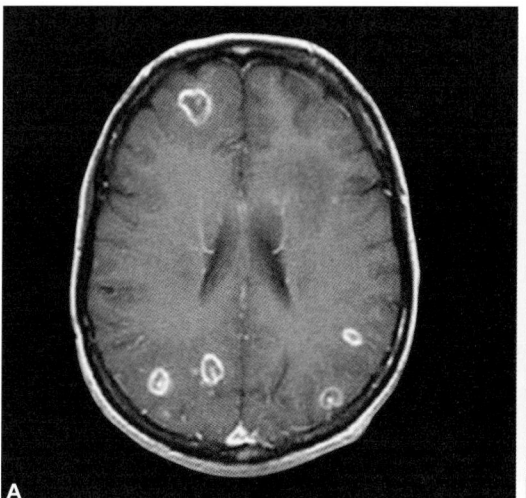 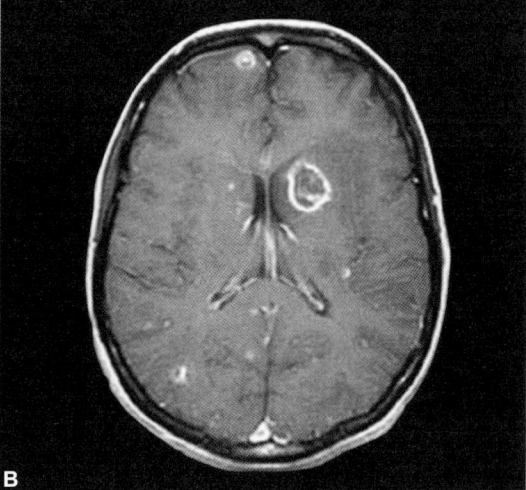

FIG. 4: T1-weighted images with gadolinium enhancement showing multiple ring enhancing lesions.

Key Points

- The commonest space occupying lesion in HIV patients is toxoplasmosis which has a predilection to involve basal ganglia and periventricular regions
- Apart from headache and seizures chorioretinitis is common in toxoplasmosis involving the central nervous system
- Pyrimethamine and sulfadiazine are treatment options which are tailored according to the immune status of the patient
- Another granulomatous parasitic infection is Chagas meningoencepahlitis which is common in HIV infected patients, caused by the parasite *Trypanosoma cruzi*. It is seen in Latin America and has not been reported from India

Fungal Infections

Cryptococcosis

Cryptococcus neoformans invades the brain when CD4 count is usually less than 100. It gains entry into the CNS from lung via blood. In the CNS it involves meninges, Virchow-Robin perivascular spaces. The inflammatory response is usually minimal and brain parenchyma is involved when CD4 count become less than 100. In the parenchyma *Cryptococcus* can cause granuloma, pseudocyst, abscess, and mixed lesions.

Clinical Features

Common clinical presentation involves headache due to involvement of Virchow-Robin spaces, signs of meningeal irritation like vomiting, seizures, altered mental status, and personality changes. Cryptococomas usually is due to *C. gatti*. Cryptococomas form in persons who are immunocompetent and involves the ependyma and choroid plexus.[33]

Diagnosis

Cryptococcal disease can be diagnosed through culture, CSF microscopy, or by cryptococcal antigen (CrAg) detection.[34] Cerebrospinal fluid CrAg is usually positive in patients with cryptococcal meningoencephalitis. Serum CrAg is usually positive in both meningeal and nonmeningeal infections and may be present weeks to months before symptom onset. Neuroimaging shows involvement of periventricular spaces and contrast enhancement is less due to lack of inflammation. Accumulation of gelatinous matter in Virchow robin spaces forms pseudocyst which causes enlargement and gives the typical soap bubble appearance. Magnetic resonance imaging shows CSF intense lesion involving the perivascular spaces which appears hypointense in T1 and hyperintense in T2. Perilesional edema may be present or absent based on the immunocompetency of the patient. Involvement of thalami and basal ganglia is common. Presence of cryptococci polysaccharide antigen in CSF and serum and demonstration of the capsule by India ink preparation aids the diagnosis.

Treatment

Treatment for cryptococcosis consists of three phases: Induction, consolidation, and maintenance therapy.[33]

- Induction therapy (for at least 2 weeks, followed by consolidation therapy). Preferred regimens: Liposomal amphotericin B 3–4 mg/kg intravenous daily plus flucytosine 25 mg/kg per oral four times a day or amphotericin B deoxycholate 0.7–1.0 mg/kg intravenous daily plus flucytosine 25 mg/kg per oral four times a day. Alternative regimens: Amphotericin B lipid complex 5 mg/kg intravenous daily plus flucytosine 25 mg/kg per oral four times a day; or liposomal amphotericin B 3–4 mg/kg intravenous daily plus fluconazole 800 mg per oral or intravenous daily or amphotericin B (deoxycholate 0.7–1.0 mg/kg intravenous daily) plus fluconazole 800 mg per oral or intravenous daily; or liposomal amphotericin B 3–4 mg/kg intravenous daily alone; or amphotericin B deoxycholate 0.7–1.0 mg/kg intravenous daily alone; or fluconazole 400 mg per oral or intravenous daily plus flucytosine 25 mg/kg per oral four times a day; or fluconazole 800 mg per oral or intravenous daily plus flucytosine 25 mg/kg

per oral four times a day; or fluconazole 1200 mg per oral or intravenous daily alone.
- Consolidation therapy (for at least 8 weeks, followed by maintenance therapy). To begin after at least 2 weeks of successful induction therapy (defined as substantial clinical improvement and a negative CSF culture after repeat LP). Drug of choice is fluconazole 400 mg per oral or intravenous once daily.

   Itraconazole 200 mg per oral twice a day is an alternate
- Maintenance therapy, preferred regimen: Fluconazole 200 mg per oral for at least 1 year
- Stopping maintenance therapy: If the following criteria are fulfilled completed initial (induction, consolidation) therapy, and at least 1 year on maintenance therapy, and remains asymptomatic from cryptococcal infection, and CD4 count ≥100 cells/μL for ≥3 months and suppressed HIV-RNA in response to effective antiretroviral therapy
- Maintenance therapy should be restarted if CD4 count declines to ≤100 cells/μL.

Key points
- Cryptococcal infection attains dangerous proportions in immune deprived patients and the typical clinical manifestations includes intense headache because of the involvement of Virchow–Robin spaces
- Cryptococcomas are seen in immunocompetent patients and it is usually secondary to *Cryptococcus gattii*
- Treatment typically involves induction, consolidation and maintenance phase and the drugs used are liposomal amphotericin and flucytosine
- Induction is for 2 weeks, consolidation is for 8 weeks and maintenance is for 1 year and for consolidation and maintenance the drug used is fluconazole

Mucormycosis

Phycomycetes are saprophytic aerobic fungi which causes rhinocerebral mucormycosis, also known as phycomycosis. The genera responsible for most cases are *Rhizopus, Absidia,* and *Mucor*. Cases of rhinocerebral mucormycosis caused by *Rhizomucor, Saksenaea, Apophysomyces,* and *Cunninghamella* species are also reported. Commonly found in bread moulds and decaying matter they become virulent in immunocompromised patients like diabetes and HIV patients where the cell mediated immunity is defective.

The fungi spreads airborne and is localized to pterygopalatine fossa. It invades neural structures, blood vessels, cartilage and bones, and thrives in acidic pH and glucose rich conditions. These conditions enable their growth and inhibits the neutrophil mediated chemotaxis.

Around 96% of patients have a risk factor and the commonest is diabetes mellitus. Apart from diabetes, immunocompromised patients secondary to burns, steroid therapy, post-transplant individuals are susceptible for rhinocerebral mucormycosis.

Clinical Features

Clinical symptoms could be because of local infiltration and spread via nerves and blood vessels.

Local spread can cause facial deformities, pain, nasal obstruction, epistaxis, periorbital pain, diplopia, and loss of vision.

Perineural spread can cause extra axial multiple cranial palsies localizing to superior orbital fissure, orbital apex, and cavernous sinus.

Spread via blood vessels involves internal carotids which can result in amaurosis fugax and ischemic strokes.

Headaches, seizures, and generalized tiredness are other clinical features.[34]

Diagnosis

Magnetic resonance imaging can detect the extent of lesion and may help in follow-up. The affected area of the brain may show diffusion restriction and will not enhance in contrast. The normal area may show contrast enhancement resulting in "black turbinate sign" seen in nasal mucosa (Fig. 5).[35]

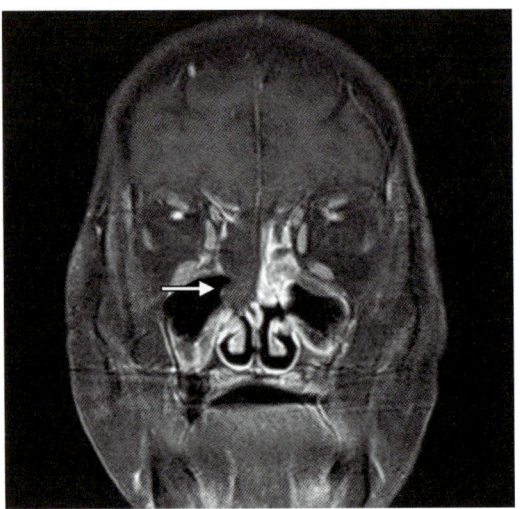

FIG. 5: Black turbinate sign-an important magnetic resonance imaging sign of mucormycosis. Fungal spores germinate to produce angioinvasive hyphae that cause infarction as they invade the nasal mucosa. This results in a 'black' area of nonenhancing mucosa which stands out against the normal enhancing mucosa.

Air fluid levels and extension to cavernous sinuses can be seen in MRI and an angiogram may show vascular occlusion usually involving the internal carotid artery.

Histopathology will confirm the diagnosis by showing the fungi.

Treatment

Correction of predisposing factors, in the form of glycemic control, withdrawing steroids, correction of acidosis etc. is done. Hyperbaric oxygen has fungistatic properties which can be tried along with granulocyte colony-stimulating factor to reconstitute the host-defense.

Systemic antifungal therapy and surgery in selected cases is mainstay in treating this life threatening disease.[34]

Amphotericin B deoxycholate remains the only licensed antifungal agent for mucormycosis. Lipid formulations of amphotericin B are considered as less toxic and equally effective. Amphotericin B lipid complex has been reported to be effective as part of a combination treatment with caspofungin.

Lipid formulation of amphotericin in the dose of 5–7.5 mg/kg/day which can be escalated up to 10 mg/kg/day is recommended for CNS involvement.

Posaconazole and isavuconazole are other treatment options in rhinocerebral mucormycosis.

Isavuconazole is effective in *Rhizopus* associated rhinocerebral mucormycosis and is FDA approved.

The duration of therapy is in months and it is guided by treatment of predisposing factors, clinical and radiological improvement.

Local debridement, drainage of abscesses and local instillation of amphotericin and reconstructive facial surgery is done in liaison with ENT, neuro, and plastic surgeons.

Despite this the fatality rate which was more than 80% before 5 years has come down to 40% for invasive mucormycosis.

Key points

- Central nervous system involvement occurs in diabetic and immunocompromised patients
- Apart from local infiltration vascular spread with involvement of internal carotid artery is very characteristic
- Magnetic resonance imaging will show the extent of involvement and black turbinate sign in the nasal mucosa
- Intravenous amphotericin or liposomal amphotericin along with local debridement are mainstay of treatment along with correction of predisposing factors

Coccidioidomycosis

Coccidioidomycosis is caused by the dimorphic soil dwelling fungus *Coccidioides immitis*. The fungus is endemic to a geographically delineated area within the United States known as the Lower Sonoran Life Zone, Mexico, and regions of Central America, which has a semiarid climate allowing the fungus to thrive.[36] Because of the same reason it is uncommon in India.

Sixty percent of patients are asymptomatic and flu like presentation is common. The disease attains dangerous proportions in nursing mothers, immunocompromised individuals, pregnant women and elderly people.

In India it is very uncommon and it is restricted to few case reports involving skin and bone.

Clinical Features

Central nervous system involvement usually presents with headache, signs of chronic meningitis, features of raised ICT due to hydrocephalus and ischemic strokes secondary to arteritis.

Cases of cerebral abscesses and dural based meningioma like lesions have also been reported.

The most common findings include hydrocephalus with ventricular enlargement, basilar meningitis, and vascular occlusion. The detection of hydrocephalus and vascular occlusion has negative prognostic implications.[37]

Treatment

Without appropriate therapy, coccidioidal meningitis is uniformly fatal and intravenous amphotericin B is not effective.

Coccidioidal meningitis treatment is tailored according to HIV status of the patient. Standard therapy in HIV negative patients consists of amphotericin B, 0.7–1 mg/kg/day, plus flucytosine, 100 mg/kg/day, for 6–10 weeks. An alternative to this regimen is amphotericin B plus 5-flucytosine for 2 weeks, followed by fluconazole 400 mg/day for a minimum of 10 weeks. Fluconazole consolidation therapy may be continued for 6–12 months, depending on the clinical status of the patient.[37]

Among patients with HIV infection and coccidioidomycosis meningitis, induction therapy with amphotericin B 0.7–1 mg/kg/day plus flucytosine 100 mg/kg/day for 2 weeks followed by fluconazole 400 mg/day for a minimum of 10 weeks is the treatment of choice. After 10 weeks of therapy, the fluconazole dosage may be reduced to 200 mg/day, depending on the patient's clinical status. Fluconazole should be continued for life. An alternative regimen for AIDS-associated cryptococcal meningitis is amphotericin B plus 5-flucytosine for 6–10 weeks, followed by fluconazole maintenance therapy. Induction therapy beginning with an azole alone is generally discouraged.

Lipid formulations of amphotericin B can be substituted for amphotericin B for patients whose renal function is impaired. Fluconazole, 400–800 mg/day plus flucytosine 100–150 mg/kg/day for 6 weeks is an alternative to the use of amphotericin B, although toxicity with this regimen is high.

Key points

- *Coccidioides immitis* associated neurological manifestations is not reported in India and more common in USA and Mexico
- Central nervous system involvement is usually in the form of meningitis, hydrocephalus and ischemic strokes
- Treatment includes parenteral amphotericin with flucytosine and in HIV patients fluconazole is given lifelong

Candidiasis

The predisposing factors for CNS candidiasis is similar to previously discussed fungal infections.

Possible ways by which *C. albicans* could penetrate the blood brain barrier are via a paracellular route by crossing between the adjacent endothelial cells, direct invasion of the endothelial cells and subsequent release from the basolateral side, indirectly via migration of the yeast infected monocytes across the endothelial barrier, or by destruction of the endothelial barrier which breaches the blood brain barrier.

Clinical Features

Clinical presentations include acute and chronic meningitis, microabcesses formation, subdural granulomas, and encephalopathy.

Diagnosis

Diagnosis of *Candida* associated meningitis should be suspected when candida is isolated in cerebrospinal fluid.

Isolation of *Candida* in any sterile liquid in patient with pleocytosis in the CSF. Blood cultures grow *Candida*.

When meningitis does not respond to conventional antibiotics and or antituberculous therapy.

Liposomal amphotericin B at a dosage of 3–5 mg/kg daily, with or without flucytosine at a dosage of 25 mg/kg 4 times daily, is recommended for the initial several weeks of treatment. Fluconazole at a dosage of 400–800 mg, i.e., 6–12 mg/kg daily is recommended as step-down therapy. Therapy should continue until all signs and symptoms abate, CSF becomes sterile and there is radiologic resolution.[38]

Removal of infected ventricular devices is recommended.

Key points
- Candida as a cause of meningitis should be considered if cerebrospinal fluid, blood or body fluids grow candida in culture and when signs of meningeal irritation is persistent despite appropriate antibiotic therapy
- Meningitis is the commonest clinical presentation and it is more common in immunocompromised patients
- Liposomal amphotericin along with flucytosine is the recommended treatment

Aspergillosis

Lungs and paranasal sinuses are primary sites of infection. *Aspergillus fumigatus* is commonest in humans followed by subspecies, *flavus*, *niger*, and *oryzae*. They are septate hyphae and spread by inhalation of spores.

Central nervous system aspergillosis is rare. CNS seeding occurs contiguously from nasal sinuses, by blood from lungs and gastrointestinal tract. In immunocompromised patients, aspergillosis usually occurs as part of a disseminated infection.

Clinical Features

The pathology of CNS aspergillosis can be classified into three forms: infarction, granulomas, and meningitis. The fungal hyphae block intracerebral blood vessels, resulting in thrombosis and subsequent infarction and clinically present as cerebrovascular accidents. The fungus can then spread beyond the vessel walls and form abscesses in the altered brain tissue.

Chronic purulent lesions can cause fibrosis and subsequent granuloma formation. Aspergillosis is the most common cause of mycotic aneurysm due to erosion of blood vessel.

Diagnosis

Microscopically, the most striking feature is the presence of the vascular invasion with thrombosis. In purulent lesions, pus is seen in the center of the abscesses with abundant polymorphs at the periphery. In patients with paranasal sinus disease orbital extension with proptosis, ocular palsies, visual deterioration, and chemosis may occur. Aspergillosis should be considered in cases manifesting with acute onset of focal neurological deficits resulting from suspected vascular or space-occupying lesions, especially in immunocompromised.

The radiological appearance of *Aspergillus* infection of the CNS is variable and depends upon the immune status of the patients. Edematous and hemorrhagic lesions, solid enhancing lesions referred to as aspergilloma or "tumoral form," abscess-like ring-like enhancing lesions, infarction, and mycotic aneurysm. Multiple areas of hypodensity on CT or hyperintensity on T2-weighted images on MRI, involving the cortex and or subcortical white matter consistent with multiple areas of infarction is a common finding in *Aspergillus* infection. The superimposed hemorrhage may be identified as hyperdensity on CT and hyperintensity on T1-weighted images (T1WI) on MR. On MRI, lesions may show areas of isointensity or low signal intensity on T2WI, which is attributed to fungal hyphae containing paramagnetic elements like manganese, iron and magnesium, but may also be related to blood breakdown products. Dural enhancement is usually seen in lesions adjacent to infected paranasal sinuses, are also seen. Diffusion-weighted imaging is valuable in early diagnosis of cerebral aspergillosis as it detects early infarction and can also be beneficial in differentiating these lesions from progressive multifocal leukoencephalopathy and neoplasm.

Elevation of glutamine–glutamate, lactate and amino acids at the central nonenhancing lesion is different from other cystic lesions. Perforating arteries are usually involved and this is due to invasion of the large walled arterial obstruction which in turn compromises blood flow to smaller perforating arteries.[39]

Treatment

- Reversal of the underlying immune deficiency: The use of colony-stimulating factors, discontinuing or reducing the dose of corticosteroids may help to restore immune function
- Antifungal therapy: Classes of antifungal drugs with good i*n vitro*/*in vivo* activity against *Aspergillus* species include:
  - Polyenes, like amphotericin
  - Azoles like voriconazole, posaconazole, isavuconazole
  - Echinocandins like caspofungin, micafungin.

Voriconazole is considered the safest and most effective antifungal drug.[39] Currently, voriconazole is the drug of choice in the treatment of confirmed invasive aspergillosis superior to amphotericin though not compared with liposomal amphotericin.

Voriconazole was successful in the treatment of CNS aspergillosis in 34% of patients, an infection previously associated with 100% mortality. Oral bioavailability of voriconazole is excellent. Therapy should be switched within a few days from the intravenous to the oral route.

The alternative drug to voriconazole is a lipid formulation of amphotericin B: either amphotericin B lipid complex or liposomal amphotericin B.

Patients generally show clinical and radiological improvement in 5–7 days. Improvement is enhanced if the underlying immune deficiency is corrected–typically, the return of neutrophils. If the immune system remains impaired, the outcome is generally poor.

Isavuconazole, a broad-spectrum antifungal agent with activity against both *Aspergillus* and *Mucor*, is indicated for the treatment of adults with invasive aspergillosis.

In case of failure of therapy with voriconazole, isavuconazole, or lipid formulations of amphotericin B, clinical deterioration is apparent in 7–10 days. Additional measures include checking serum concentrations of voriconazole (2 μg/mL or greater for efficacy), switching from voriconazole to lipid formulations of amphotericin B and/or an echinocandin, or adding an echinocandin to therapy with voriconazole for potential synergy. Combination therapy an azole antifungal plus an echinocandin may be more effective than monotherapy with an azole.

For salvage therapy, multiple drugs have been used simultaneously as a desperate measure with a success rate of about 40%.

> **Key points**
> - Central nervous system aspergillosis is rare but can cause meningitis, granulomas and ischemic strokes in appropriate setting
> - Mycotic aneurysms are usually due to aspergillosis
> - Vascular spread is noted and strokes corresponding to perforating arteries are common
> - Voriconazole and liposomal amphotericin either alone or in combination with azoles or echinocandins improves outcome

Immunological Causes

Relapsing Polychondritis

Relapsing polychondritis is a rare autoimmune disorder which usually involves cartilages and neurological involvement occurs only in 3% of patients.

Clinical Features

- Meningitis, pachymeningitis, cranial nerve palsies, strokes, limbic encephalitis, and seizures are common clinical presentation
- The meningeal inflammation is usually a granuloma
- Among the cranial nerves, second cranial nerve is most often involved
- Vasculitis of small and median sized vessels results in strokes and encephalitis
- McAdam's diagnostic criteria is applied for the diagnosis of relapsing polychondritis.[40-42]

Three of the following six, are necessary for diagnosis:
1. Bilateral auricular chondritis
2. Nonerosive seronegative inflammatory polyarthritis
3. Nasal chondritis
4. Ocular inflammation
5. Respiratory tract chondritis
6. Audiovestibular damage.

Though biopsy is confirmatory it is performed only if the diagnosis is in doubt.

Treatment

Steroids are the main stay of treatment. In CNS meningitis, parenteral steroids followed by prednisone 20–60 mg/day is administered in the acute phase and is tapered to 5–25 mg/day for maintenance. Higher doses of steroids also may be given during flare ups. Most patients require a low daily dose of prednisone for maintenance.

Dapsone, methotrexate, cyclophosphamide, azathioprine, and cyclosporin A are other drugs used to prevent relapses and maintain remission.

Methotrexate at 7.5 mg/week along with steroids prevents relapses and also decreases the dose requirement of steroids. Methotrexate can be increased up to 22.5 mg/week.[4]

Key points
- Neurological involvement in only 2%percent of patients with relapsing polychondritis
- Meningitis and among cranial nerves second cranial nerve is common clinical presentation
- Diagnosis is clinical and McAdam's clinical criteria is useful
- Steroids are used for acute attacks and methotrexate is favored as disease modifying drug along with low dose steroids

Neuro-Behçet's Disease

Behçet's is a multisystem disease secondary to inflammatory perivasculitis.

Knapp first reported neuro-Behçet's disease in 1941.

Neurological involvement occurs in 4–49% of patients with Behçet's disease and the disease is more common in Mediterranean population.

Clinical Features

Parenchymal and nonparenchymal are two categories of CNS involvement in Behçet's.

Subacute meningoencephalitis accounts for 75% of cases in parenchymal neuro-Behçet's.

Lower cranial nerve involvement, bipyramidal and pancerebellar involvement pertaining to brain stem is common presentation.

A progressive form of the disease representing 10% of cases of neuro-Behçet's, includes, a worsening subcortical dementia, along with ataxia.

Symptoms and signs suggestive of cerebral hemispheric involvement include encephalopathy, hemiparesis, hemisensory loss, seizures, language disturbance, and mental changes like cognitive dysfunction and psychosis. Spinal cord involvement include pyramidal signs in the limbs, sensory level, and autonomic disturbance. The myelopathy can have a severe primary progressive course, a secondary progressive course after initial attacks, or an acute attack with severe residual disability.

Lastly, asymptomatic parenchymal neuro-Behçet's is diagnosed if there are no neurological symptoms, but neurological signs on examination.[43]

Epilepsy has been observed in 2–5 % of patients. Generalized, partial and epilepsia partialis continua have all been reported.

Necrotic lesions mimicking a tumor have also been reported with a predilection to brainstem, diencephalon, basal ganglia, and internal capsule.

Isolated meningitis and optic neuropathy are syndromes secondary to Behçet's.

Nonparenchymal involvement includes ischemic strokes, venous strokes, and aneurysm formation.

Though superior sagittal sinus is commonly involved, deep system involving vein of Rosenthal is characteristic.

Psychiatric, cognitive disturbance, headache mimicking migraine and tension type headache are also noted.

Diagnosis

Diagnosis is clinical. The HLA-B51 is commonly associated with the disease. Raised cell count and protein are noted in CSF. Similarly interleukins-6, 8, TNF, and interferons are noted, but all this is not specific.

Magnetic resonance imaging aids the diagnosis and it is not specific. The most common site of involvement is brainstem and the next most common sites are basal ganglia and white matter.

Treatment

Intravenous methylprednisolone: 1g intravenous daily for 3-5 days followed by oral prednisone 0.5-1 mg/kg/day is given for the acute attack followed by oral taper which is done slowly over a period of 2-3 months. Azathioprine, cyclophosphamide, chlorambucil, thalidomide, and methotrexate are the common immunosuppressant drugs used to prevent flare ups. Azathioprine and methotrexate are the preferred drugs.

Key points
- Neuro-Behçet's occurs in 4-45% of patients with Behçet's disease
- Parenchymal and nonparenchymal involvement are two categories of brain involvement
- Subacute meningoencephalitis, brain stem involvement, cranial neuropathies, seizures, and myelopathy are due to parenchymal involvement
- Strokes, arterial, and venous and headache are nonparenchymal involvement of the disease
- Diagnosis is clinical and steroids are used during acute attacks

Neurological Manifestations of Antineutophilic Cytoplasmic Antibody Associated Diseases

Three systemic autoimmune diseases: Granulomatosis with polyangitis, microscopic polyangiitis, and eosinophilic granulomatosis with polyangiitis are three antineutophilic cytoplasmic antibody (ANCA) disorders which share common pathogenesis in causing small and medium vessel vasculitis and granuloma formation. Granulomatosis with polyangiitis and eosinophilic granulomatosis with polyangiitis were previously called as Wegner's granulomatosis and Churg–Strauss syndrome.

Incidence ranging from 15 to 25 per 1 million occurs in the general population.

Respiratory tract and kidneys are frequently involved but CNS involvement is common and well documented.

Clinical Features

Peripheral nervous system involvement is marked by mononeuritis multiplex most frequently in eosinophilic granulomatosis with polyangiitis.

Peroneal, tibial, ulnar, and median nerves are commonly affected.

Symmetrical peripheral neuropathy and mononeuropathies also occur.

Central nervous system involvement occurs in 5-15% of ANCA positive patients and common clinical presentations are headache, cranial nerve involvement, meningitis, pachymeningitis, neuropsychiatric manifestations, vestibular syndrome, ischemic and hemorrhagic strokes. Pituitary involvement has also been reported.

Pachymeningitis can involve the spinal cord also.

Apart from detection of the specific antibodies and clinical manifestations MRI can aid in the diagnosis but it is not specific. Diffuse white matter changes and pachymeningitis can be detected in MRI.[44-46]

Treatment

Treatment regimens include induction of remission and maintenance phase.

Induction of remission is usually for three months and maintenance is for 24 months.

Standard initial therapy starts with high-dose corticosteroids. Prednisone, 1 mg/kg for approximately 1 month. It is then tapered and an additional immunosuppressive agent such as cyclophosphamide 15 mg/kg adjusted to age and renal function, preferably intravenous pulses every 2-3 weeks. Maintenance therapy is based on low-dose corticosteroids, azathioprine or methotrexate.

Leflunomide, should be avoided in cases with neurological manifestation because of neurotoxic side effects.

Rituximab and plasmapheresis can be tried in refractory cases.[45,47]

> **Key points**
> - Antineutophilic cytoplasmic antibody positive diseases can involve central and peripheral nervous system and eosinophilic granulomatosis with angitis commonly causes mononeuritis multiplex
> - Detection of appropriate antibodies in a clinical setting gives the correct diagnosis
> - Steroids for induction of remission and low dose steroids along with judicious use of steroid sparing drugs are treatment options

Neurosarcoidosis

Sarcoidosis is an idiopathic non caseating granulomatous disease involving various systems. Among which neurosarcoidosis accounts for 5–13% of cases. It may present as isolated neurosarcoidosis or with multisystem involvement.[48,49]

Neurosarcoidosis is thought to develop from an initial granulomatous inflammatory meningitis. These exudates from subarachnoid space via Virchow–Robins space reaches the brain parenchyma causing granulomas in brain. It may also be a consequence of perineural spread from sinonasal sarcoidosis. In peripheral nerves granulomas accumulate in perinerium and endoneurium leading to axonal neuropathy.

The characteristic lesion of sarcoidosis is a discrete, compact, noncaseating granulomatous epithelioid cell granuloma which has predominant CD4 lymphocytes in the central region and CD8 in the periphery.

Clinical Features

The clinical manifestation may differ depending on the localization of the inflammatory process. Cranial nerve neuropathy is the most common manifestation and facial nerve is the most frequently involved among the cranial nerves. Facial nerve palsy along with bilateral parotid gland enlargement, anterior uveitis and fever is known as Heerfordt syndrome. Eighth nerve dysfunction due to sarcoidosis typically presents as sensorineural hearing loss. Optic neuropathy is most common presentation according to some and it may be unilateral or bilateral. Meningeal infiltration preferentially involves the basal leptomeninges and may cause aseptic meningitis which may mimic cryptococcal meningitis. It may present with neuropsychiatric manifestations like depression 60–66% and neuroendocrinological dysfunction like diabetes insipidus, hypothalamic dysfunction and amenorrhea-galactorrhea syndrome. It may also present as headache (17–48%) hydrocephalus (38%), seizures, peripheral neuropathy and myopathy. Neurosarcoidosis may mimic multiple sclerosis and progressive multifocal encephalopathy. The signs of spinal cord sarcoidosis mimics those of spinal cord tumor or meningomyelitis. Radiculopathy is a rare manifestation of sarcoidosis. The most common type of peripheral neuropathy in sarcoidosis is a symmetric axonal polyneuropathy.

The diagnostic criteria proposed by Zajicek with levels of certainity are:[50] (i) Possible neurosarcoidosis–clinical presentation suggestive of neurosarcoidosis with exclusion of other possible diagnoses; (ii) probable–above plus laboratory support for CNS inflammation (elevated CSF protein and/or cells, oligoclonal bands, MRI evidence compatible with neurosarcoidosis); (iii) definite neurosarcoidosis–above plus the presence of positive nervous system histology.[48]

Diagnosis

Magnetic resonance imaging brain with gadolinium enhancement is considered the most sensitive noninvasive test for neurosarcoidosis. The most common finding is leptomeningeal involvement seen in form of nodules or plaques which reveal focal or diffuse thickening with contrast enhancement. Cerebrospinal fluid study may show pleocytosis, oligoclonal bands. Electroencephalography may show focal or generalized slowing. Bronchoalveolar lavage may show increased CD4:CD8 ratio.

Angiotensin converting enzyme level may be elevated in 65% of patients. Tissue biopsy reveals non caseating granulomas. Gallium 67 citrate scan are positive only in 45% of patients.

Treatment

Corticosteroids are the first line drugs for treatment. Oral prednisolone at 40–80 mg/day. In severe cases intravenous corticosteroids can be given. The second line of treatment includes steroid-sparing drugs like methotrexate, cyclosporine, cyclophosphamide, chlorambucil and mycophenolate mofetil. The other options are Infliximab (TNF-alpha blocker), chloroquine, radiation therapy (dose 20–25 Gy).

> **Key points**
> - Neurological manifestations occurs in 5–12% of patients of sarcoidosis
> - Neurological features are protean and can involve cranial nerves, meninges, cognition, brain parenchyma, and spinal cord
> - Contrast enhanced magnetic resonance imaging, bronchoalveolar lavage, cerebrospinal fluid analysis, serum angiotensin converting enzyme levels and biopsy aids in diagnosis
> - Steroids is the cornerstone in treatment

Neoplastic Granulomas

Langerhans Cell Histiocytosis

Langerhans cell histiocytosis is a rare disease secondary to an abnormal deposit of dendritic cells in different tissues similar to Langerhans cells.

Neurodegenerative and tumors are two clinical presentations of neurologic Langerhans cell histiocytosis.

Neurodegenerative is second commonest presentation and has a progressive course that varies in severity. It is not usually the initial or only manifestation of the disease, but usually appear several years after the initial diagnosis.

Neurodegenerative symptoms could be asymptomatic or manifest with ataxia, gait disturbances, spastic paraparesis, dysarthria, and cognitive regression.

Space occupying lesions presenting like a tumor is the common presentation and frequently involves the hypothalamic pituitary axis. It can also involve the brainstem and cerebellum.

Involvement of hypothalamic pituitary axis causes diabetes insipidus.

According to the "Histiocyte Society", the radiological manifestations of Langerhans cell histiocytosis in the CNS can be classified into:
- Intracranial extra-axial lesions
  - *Hypothalamic-pituitary axis*: "Loss of bright spot', is the lack of the physiologic hyperintense signal of the posterior pituitary on T1-weighted image which correlates with the loss of antidiuretic hormone containing granules. Loss of bright spot sign is shown in fig. 6. Infiltrating masses in this region, can present like a tumor
  - *Other locations*: Meninges-causing enhancement with contrast.

Choroid plexus can cause obstruction and hydrocephalus. It mimics a choroid plexus papilloma.

Pineal gland-cystic enlargement of the gland can be seen in the MRI.

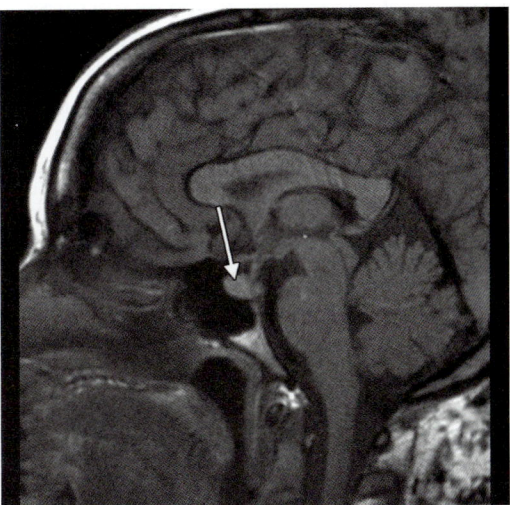

FIG. 6: MRI imaging of brain revealed loss of posterior pituitary bright spot.

- Intracranial intra-axial lesions
  - *Intraparenchymal lesions*: They manifest as rounded masses with abnormal signals that are iso to hypointense to gray matter on the T1 and hyperintense on T2WI. These areas show intense contrast enhancement and have well demarcated edges and can produce mass effect
  - *Neurodegenerative disease*: Degeneration of cerebellum especially involving the dentate nucleus gives the "butter fly pattern" in the coronal cuts, with T2 hypointensity and T2 hyperintensity.
- Leukoencephalopathy-like pattern manifest as poorly defined T2 hyperintense areas in the cerebral periventricular white matter, pons and cerebellar white matter, without mass effect or contrast enhancement. Cerebellar and supratentorial atrophy is one of the most nonspecific findings described in neurological Langerhans cell histiocytosis.[51,52]

Diagnosis

Diagnosis of Langerhans cell histiocytosis is made following a biopsy and microscopic examination of the affected tissue. A definitive diagnosis requires the immune histochemical identification of the presence of Langerhans cells by cell surface CD1a or is made by the presence of cells with Birbeck granules by electron microscopy. Paraffin-embedded specimens can now identify CD1a surface antigen making electron microscopy unnecessary. If the biopsy is positive for Langerhans cell histiocytosis, skeletal X-ray survey with skull X-ray series and bone scan are done to assess the extent of the disease. Magnetic resonance imaging of brain showing butterfly pattern.

Treatment

There is no established, widely agreed-upon treatment of Langerhans cell histiocytosis in general. It depends upon the individual patient and the extent and areas of involvement. Treatment protocol for disseminated or multisystem disease involves two major approaches a conservative approach with minimal chemotherapy along with steroids for low-risk diseases and an intensive chemotherapy complimented with low dose radiotherapy or surgery for high-risk diseases. Some patients have had success with vinblastine and steroids, while others have benefited from limited surgery along with drug therapy. Other chemotherapy agents such as vincristine, cytosine arabinoside in combination have been found useful.[53] Low-dose external beam radiation can benefit in an individual patient. Some patients may have limited involvement, which does not progress to other areas and may not need systemic treatment.

> **Key points**
> - Langerhans cell histiocytosis can involve neuraxis in two forms tumorous and neurodegenerative forms
> - Tumorous presentation is common involving the hypothalamic pituitary axis clinically presenting as diabetes insipidus
> - Two characteristic MRI features are loss of bright spot in the posterior pituitary and butterfly pattern in cerebellum
> - Biopsy demonstrating CD1a antigen in Langerhans cell and Birbeck granules in electron microscopy gives the definitive diagnosis
> - For neurological Langerhans cell histiocytosis conservative and intensive approach as outlined in text is practiced
> - Pyogenic granuloma and benign fibrous histiocytoma are two other nontuberculous granulomatous conditions involving brain very rarely

CONCLUSION

Nontuberculous granulomas has a great diversity in etiology as well as in clinical presentations. Different infectious granulomatous diseases have different areas of endemicity and poses a diagnostic challenge. Neuroimaging techniques often don't give the correct diagnosis. Though histopathology will give the definitive diagnosis it cannot be done in all patients. Clinical clues, geographic location and serological tests for antibodies against the pathogens are important aids in diagnosing nontuberculous and noncysticercus granulomas. Constant migration of population and air travel helps in disseminating infection to different corners of the world which further makes things difficult for the clinician. Once the diagnosis is achieved treatment is tailored according to the etiology. The important thing to bear in mind is though granulomas have varied etiology the most common cause however is infection.

REFERENCES

1. Williams GT, Williams WJ. Granulomatous inflammation: A review. J Clin Pathol. 1983;36(7):723-33.
2. Zumla A, James DG. Granulomatous infections: Etiology and classification. Clin Infect Dis. 1996;23: 146-58.
3. Mishra NK, Goulatia RK, Khosla A. Granulomas of the brain. In: du Boulay G., Molyneux A. Moseley I. (eds). Proceedings of the XIV Symposium Neuroradiologicum. Springer, Berlin, Heidelberg. 1991.
4. Rajeev KR, Lyme disease outbreak in Wayanad, TNN, The Times of India [newspaper on the Internet]. March 2, 2013. Available:http://timesofindia. indiatimes. com/city/kozhikode/Lyme-disease-outbreak-in Wayanad/articleshow/18758675. cms?referral=PM
5. Jairath V, Sehrawat M, Jindal N, et al. Lyme disease in Haryana, India. Indian J Dermatol Venereol Leprol. 2014;80:320-3.
6. Hildenbrand P, Craven DE, Jones R, et al. Nemeskal Lyme neuroborreliosis: Manifestations of a rapidly emerging zoonosis. AJNR Am J Neuroradiol. 2009;30(6):1079-87.
7. Michael T. Melia, Paulg. Auwaerter, New England journal of medicine 2016:374:1277-1278/March 2016.
8. Guven T, Ugurlu K, Ergonul O, et al. Neurobrucellosis: Clinical and diagnostic features. Clin Infect Dis. 2013;56(10):1407-12.
9. Conde-Sendin MA, Amela-Peris R, Aladro-Benito Y, et al. Current clinical spectrum of neurosyphilis in immunocompetent patients. EurNeurol. 2004;52:29-35.
10. Seeley WW, Venna N. Neurosyphilis presenting with gummatous oculomotor nerve palsy. J Neurol Neurosurg Psychiatry. 2004;75:789.
11. Holland B, Perrett L, Mills C. Meningovascular syphilis: CT and MR findings. Radiology. 1986;158:439-42.
12. Gallego J, Soriano G, Zubieta JL, et al. Magnetic resonance angiography in meningovascular syphilis. Neuroradiology. 1994;36:208-9.
13. Corr P, Bhigjee A, Lockhat F. Oculomotor nerve root enhancement in meningovascular syphilis, Journal of Clinical Radiology, March 2004,Vol.59, 294-296.
14. Mara CM, Maxwell CL, Stacy L, et al. Barnett cerebrospinal fluid abnormalitites in patients with syphilis: Association with clinical and laboratory features. J Infect Dis. 2004;189(3):369-76.
15. Khosla VK, Banerjee AK, Chopra JS. Intracranial actinomycoma with osteomyelitis simulating meningioma. J Neurosurg.1984;60:204-7.
16. Moniruddin AB, Begum H, Nahar K. Actinomycosis: An update. Medicine Today 2010;22:437.
17. Mohindra S, Savardekar A, Rane S. Intracranial actinomycosis: Varied clinical and radiologic presentations in two cases. Neurol India. 2012;60:325-7.
18. Reibel F, Cambau E, Aubry A. Update on the epidemiology, diagnosis, and treatment of leprosy. Médecine et Maladies Infectieuses. 2015;45(9):383-93.
19. Scollard DM, Adams LB, Gillis TP, et al. The continuing challenges of leprosy. Clin Microbiol Rev. 2006;19(2):338-81.
20. Ghosh SN, Kesharwani A, Chaudhuri S, et al. Rhinoscleroma with intracranial extension: A rare case. 2016;64(3):549-52.
21. Chomel BB .Cat-scratch disease and bacillary angiomatosis. 1996;15(3);1061-73.
22. Hansmann Y, DeMartino S, Piémont Y,et al. Diagnosis of cat scratch disease with Detection of Bartonella henselae by PCR: A study of patients with lymph node enlargement Arch Neurol. 2005;62(6):1008-10.
23. Betting LE, Pirani C Jr, de Souza Queiroz L, et al. Seizures and cerebral schistosomiasis. Arch Neurol. 2005;62(6):1008-10.
24. Wan H, Masataka H, Lei T, et al. Magnetic resonance imaging and cerebrospinal fluid immunoassay in the diagnosis of cerebral schistosomiasis: Experience in southwest China. Trans R Soc Trop Med Hyg. 2009;103(10):1059-61.
25. Singh TS, Sugiyama H, Rangsiruji A. Paragonimus & paragonimiasis in India. Indian J Med Res. 2012;136(2):192-204.
26. Zhang JS, Huan Y, Sun L. MRI features of CNS pediatric cerebral paragonimasis in the active stage. J Magn Reson Imaging. 2006;23(4):569-73.
27. John DT. Primary amebic meningoencephalitis and the biology of Naegleria fowleri. Annu Rev Microbiol. 1982;36:101-23.
28. Schumacher DJ, Tien RD, Lane K. Neuroimaging findings in rare amebic infections of the central nervous system. AJNR Am J Neuroradiol. 1995;16:930-5.
29. Healy JF. Balamuthia amebic encephalitis: radiographic and pathologic findings. AJNR Am J Neuroradiol. 2002;23:486-9.
30. Gupta S, Desai K, Goel A. Intracranial hydatid cyst : A report of five cases and review of literature.1999;3:214-7.
31. Ramsey RG, Gean AD. Neuroimagingof AIDS. I. Central nervous system toxoplasmosis. Neuroimaging Clin N Am. 1997;7:171-86.
32. Ionita C, Wasay M, Balos L, et al. MR imaging in toxoplasmosis encephalitis after bone marrow transplantation: Paucity of enhancement despite fulminant disease. AJNR Am J Neuroradiol. 2004;25:270-3.
33. Saag MS, Graybill RJ, Larsen RA, et al. Practice guidelines for the management of cryptococcal disease. Infectious Diseases Society of America. Clin Infect Dis. 2000;30(4):710-8.

34. Richardson M, Koukila-Kahkola P, Shankland G, et al. Rhizopus, Rhizomucor, Absidia, and other agents of systemic and subcutaneous zygomycoses Manual of Clinical Microbiology. 9th ed. Washington, DC: American Society of Microbiology; 2007.
35. Safder S, Carpenter JS, Roberts TD, et al. The "Black Turbinate" sign: An early MR imaging finding of nasal mucormycosis. AJNR Am J Neuroradiol. 2010;31(4):771-4..
36. Brown J, Benedict K, Park BJ, et al. Coccidioidomycosis: Epidemiology. Clin Epidemiol. 2013;5:185-97.
37. Mathisen G, Shelub A, Truong J, et al. Coccidiodal meningitis clinical presentation and management in fluconazole era. Medicine (Baltimore). 2010;89(5): 251-84.
38. Pappas PG, Kauffman CA, Andes D, et al. Clinical practice guidelines for the management of candidiasis: 2009 update by the Infectious Diseases Society of America. Clin Infect Dis. 2009;48(5):503-35.
39. Rhunke S, Kofla G, Otto K, et al. CNS Aspergillosis: Recognition diagnosis and management. CNS Drugs. 2007;21(8):659-76.
40. Sosada B, Loza K, Bialo-Wojcicka E. Relapsing polychondritis. Case Rep Dermatol Med. 2014;2014:791951. (45).
41. Letko E, Zafirakis P, Baltatzis S, et al. Relapsing polychondritis: A clinical review. Semin Arthritis Rheum. 2002;31(6):384-95.
42. Fernando Kemta Lekpa, Xavier Chevalier, Refractory relapsing polychondritis: challenges and solutions, Open Access Rheumatol. 2018; 10: 1–11.
43. Tunc T, Ortapamuk H, Naldoken S, et al. Subclinical neurological involvement in Behcet's disease. 2006;54(4):408-11.
44. Olsen KD, Neel HB 3rd, Deremee RA, et al. Nasal manifestations of allergic granulomatosis and angitis (Churg-Strauss syndrome). Otolaryngol Head Neck Surg. 1980;88(1): 85-9.
45. Abril A, Calamia KT, Cohen MD. The Churg Strauss syndrome (allergic granulomatous angiitis): review and update. Semin Arthritis Rheum 2003; 33(2):106–14.
46. Bacciu A, Bacciu S, Mercante G, et al. Ear, nose and throat manifestations of Churg-Strauss syndrome. Acta Otolaryngol. 2006;126(5):503-9.
47. Gottschlich S, Ambrosch P, Kramkowski D, et al. Head and neck manifestations of Wegener's granulomatosis. Rhinology. 2006;44(4):227-33.
48. Nozaki K, Judson MA. Neurosarcoidosis: Clinical manifestations, diagnosis and treatment. 2012;41: e331-48.
49. Stern BJ, Krumholz A, Johns C, et al. Sarcoidosis and its neurological manifestations Arch Neurol. 1985;42:909-17.
50. Richard T.Ibitoye, A.Wilkins and N.J.Scolding, Neurosarcoidosis: A clinical approach to diagnosis and manangement, Journal of Neurology, 2017, 264(5), 1023-1028.
51. Komp DM. Historical perspectives of Langerhans cell histiocytosis. Hematol Oncol Clin North Am. 1987;1(1):9-21.
52. Merad M, Ginhoux F, Collin M. Origin, homeostasis and function of Langerhans cells and other langerin-expressing dendritic cells. Nat Rev Immunol. 2008;8(12):935-47.
53. Allen CE, Flores R, Rauch R, et al Neurodegenerative central nervous system Langerhans cell histiocytosis and coincident hydrocephalus treated with vincristine/cytosine arabinoside. Pediatr Blood Cancer. 2010;54(3):416-23.

CHAPTER 5

Management of Normal Pressure Hydrocephalus

Sarala Govindarajan, Harish Jayakumar, Shunmuga S Kanthimathinathan, R Lakshminarasimhan Ranganathan

INTRODUCTION

Normal pressure hydrocephalus (NPH) is a disorder of cerebrospinal fluid (CSF) absorption that results in the development of characteristic triad of symptoms (hakim's triad)—Dementia, urinary incontinence, and gait disturbance. This condition was first described by Hakim and Adams in 1965. Despite several advancements in the field of neurology, this entity is still a disease that can be included in the differential diagnosis of several other diseases presenting with the same symptoms. This article summarizes the approach to diagnosis and management of NPH.

PATHOPHYSIOLOGY

The CSF is normally produced in the choroid plexus within the lateral and fourth ventricles, from which it passes through the foramina of Luschka and Magendie and enters the cisterna magna, then bathing the superior cerebral convexities in the subarachnoid space, and finally being absorbed by the arachnoid granulations, mainly in the superior sagittal sinus. Normal pressure hydrocephalus is a disorder of absorption, not excess formation.[1] Whether from an established or unknown cause, the arachnoid granulations fail to maintain their baseline removal of CSF, often secondary to fibrosis and scarring that obscure absorptive interfaces. A pressure gradient develops between the fluid in the subarachnoid space surrounding the brain and the ventricular system. The differential pressures eventually lead to decreased CSF production and the setting of a higher, yet still normal, baseline pressure.[2] This new pressure distends the ventricles, stretching surrounding nerve fibers and compressing the periventricular parenchyma. This encroachment on brain tissue by enlarged ventricles impinges on the caliber of arterioles and capillaries, often resulting in ischemia.[3] In idiopathic normal pressure hydrocephalus (INPH), clinical deterioration is probably due to impaired periventricular blood flow associated to interstitial edema, ependyma disruption, microvascular infarctions, gliosis, and neuronal degeneration.[4] Neuronal injury may result from mechanical stretching of periventricular tissue by the enlarging ventricles, impairment of blood brain barrier, reduced CSF turnover and disturbed elimination of neurotoxic substances such as β-amyloid, tau-protein, and pro-inflammatory cytokines.[5,6]

CLINICAL SYMPTOMS

All components of the triad is seen in 50–75% of cases. The combination of gait and cognitive disturbances occurs in 80–95%, and urinary incontinence alone in 50–75% of cases.[7] In classical cases, gait disturbance is the first and most ominous sign, followed by memory disturbance or mild dementia, psychomotor retardation, apathy, parkinsonian features and, later on, urinary urgency or incontinence.

Gait Disturbance

In the later stages and NPH in its full blown state, the prime sign is a broad-based, short-stepping, magnetic gait with ignition failure as start hesitation and increased unsteadiness on turning, with frequent falls. The gait of INPH is common with the features of gait in Parkinson disease, progressive supranuclear palsy, and cerebellar ataxia. The ignition failure attributed to frontal dysfunction is very similar and in most cases is considered as apraxia of gait.[8] The term "gait apraxia" has been considered incongruous in INPH, since these patients may be able to perform or imitate walking movements without any difficulty when supported or lying down.[9] Hence, this gait disturbance has been attributed to a disconnection between frontal lobe, basal ganglia circuitry and therefore resulting in uninhibited antigravity reflexes with cocontraction of agonist and antagonists during walking.[9,10]

Cognitive Deficits

The impairment in cognition is predominantly of subcortical type with patients having difficulty in attention, memory, executive functions and have apathy and psychomotor slowing. Cortical signs like apraxia, agnosia; though not typical, are very rare in NPH. Dementia if present is usually mild, and if it's the most prominent feature and more severe, the probable diagnosis is Alzheimer's disease (AD) and not NPH. Dementia is usually accompanied with psychiatric symptoms such as irritability, emotional instability, increased fatigability, impairment in concentration, and in severe cases there can be emotional and motivational blunting. These constitute an astheno-emotional syndrome.[11,12]

Urinary Incontinence

The last to present is urinary disturbances, but at early stages urinary frequency and urgency may be present. Stretching of periventricular nerve fibers with sequential loss of voluntary supraspinal control of bladder contractions is responsible for the presentation of urinary symptoms.[13] The frequent symptoms include urgency/frequency and incontinence.[14] As the disease progresses, even fecal incontinence may occur.

CLASSIFICATION OF NORMAL PRESSURE HYDROCEPHALUS[15]

Newer classification for NPH has been proposed based on the etiology. If the patient with NPH had previous childhood acquired illness like, subarachnoid hemorrhage or meningitis or developmental anomalies like Blake's pouch cyst, symptoms may manifest late in the adulthood with features of NPH. Such patients are classified to be secondary NPH. Primary or Idiopathic NPH is defined when no recognizable etiology has been found (Flowchart 1). They are further

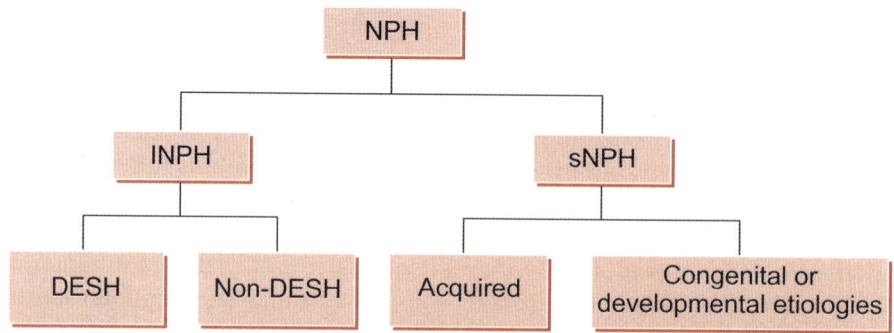

DESH, Disproportionately enlarged subarachnoid space hydrocephalus; INPH, idiopathic normal pressure hydrocephalus; NPH, normal pressure hydrocephalus; sNPH, secondary normal pressure hydrocephalus.

FLOWCHART 1: Classification of normal pressure hydrocephalus.

classified into disproportionately enlarged subarachnoid space hydrocephalus (DESH) and non-DESH INPH based on the presence or absence of DESH. Disproportionately enlarged subarachnoid space hydrocephalus is defined as disproportionately enlarged subarachnoid space hydrocephalus. Previously studies in INPH have demonstrated magnetic resonance imaging (MRI) findings of narrowed CSF spaces in the high convexity and midline, and increased CSF spaces in the Sylvian fissure and basal cistern. The importance of DESH in the pathophysiology of NPH remains to be clarified.[15]

DIAGNOSTIC CRITERIA FOR IDIOPATHIC NORMAL PRESSURE HYDROCEPHALUS[15]

- Possible INPH meets all of the following five features:
  - Onset of symptoms in age >60 years or older
  - One or more of clinical triad: gait disturbance, cognitive impairment, and urinary incontinence
  - Ventricular dilatation (Evans' index >0.3)
  - Above symptoms and findings not attributable to any other neurological illness
  - No prior history of preceding illness possibly causing ventricular dilation, including subarachnoid hemorrhage, meningitis, head injury, congenital hydrocephalus, and aqueductal stenosis.
- Possible INPH supportive features:
  - Small stride, shuffling, instability during walking, and increase of instability on turning
  - Slow progression of symptoms; an undulating course, including temporal discontinuation of development and exacerbation of symptoms
  - Gait disturbance is the most ominous feature, followed by cognitive impairment and urinary incontinence
  - Cognitive impairment is demonstrable on subjective cognitive testing
  - Enlargement of Sylvian fissures and basal cistern
  - Other neurological diseases, including Parkinson's disease, AD, and cerebrovascular diseases, may coexist; however, all such diseases should be mild
  - Periventricular changes are not essential
  - Measurement of cerebral blood flow is useful for differentiation from other dementias
  - Possible INPH with MRI support: Includes the condition satisfying the requirements for possible INPH, with MRI showing narrowing of the sulci and subarachnoid spaces over the high convexity/midline surface (DESH).
- Probable INPH meets all of the following three features:
  - Meets the requirements for possible INPH
  - CSF pressure of 200 mmH$_2$O or less with normal CSF content
  - One of the following three investigational features:
    - Neuroimaging features of narrowing of the sulci and subarachnoid spaces over the high convexity/midline surface (DESH) under the presence of gait disturbance
    - Improvement of symptoms after CSF tap test
    - Improvement of symptoms after CSF drainage test.
- Definite INPH Improvement of symptoms after the shunt procedure.

IMAGING

Computed Tomography and Magnetic Resonance Imaging

Imaging using computed tomography (CT) and MRI may show ventricular dilatation (Fig. 1). Dilatation of subarachnoid spaces in the Sylvian fissures and over the ventral surface below and narrowing of subarachnoid spaces over the high cerebral convexity and medial surface.[15] Disappearance of sulci in the dorsoposterior

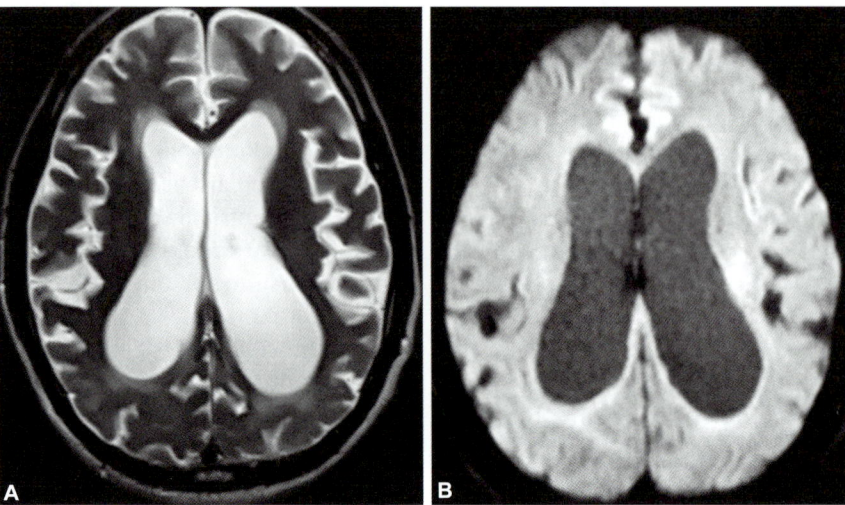

FIG. 1: Dilated ventricles with Evans ratio more than 0.3. Normal pressure hydrocephalus.

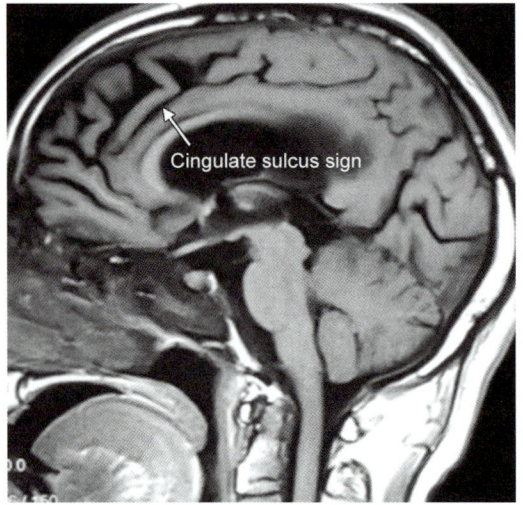

FIG. 2: Cingulate sulcus sign: Posterior half of the cingulate sulcus is narrower than the anterior half.

part of the brain along with tight high convexity subarachnoid spaces on two sequential coronal sections of T1 weighted MRI is considered a hallmark for NPH.[16] This tight high convexity subarachnoid space can reliably differentiate INPH from AD with high sensitivity and specificity.[15] This finding is due to retention of CSF in subarachnoid spaces in the Sylvian fissure and below them, resulting in decrease in the subarachnoid spaces on the dorsal surface. This leads to disproportionate enlargement of subarachnoid space between superior and inferior spaces, hence the term DESH.[16] Cingulate Sulcus sign (Fig. 2)–a highly sensitive and specific sign for NPH is seen in the sagittal MRI sections through the posterior commissure.[17] The posterior half of the cingulate sulcus is narrower than the anterior half on sagittal MRI sections, whereas in normal individuals the anterior half is usually narrower or equal to the posterior half of the sulcus. Both these signs can reliably differentiate AD from INPH. Periventricular ischemic changes as a result of ischemia due to stretching can be seen.[15] There is inverse correlation between response to CSF tap test and degree of white matter changes.[18]

Imaging Diagnostic Criteria[19]

Recommendations from International Guidelines have been implemented for the diagnosis of NPH and selection of shunt-responsive patients:
- Enlargement of Ventricles not entirely attributable to cerebral atrophy or congenital enlargement (Evans' index >0.3)
- No macroscopic obstruction to CSF flow
- At least one of the following supportive features:

- Temporal horn enlargement not attributable to hippocampus atrophy
- Callosal angle of 40° or greater
- Evidence of altered brain water content, including periventricular signal changes on CT and MRI not attributable to microvascular ischemic changes or demyelination
- An aqueductal or fourth ventricular flow void on MRI.

The following features are included in the Japanese INPH Guidelines:[15]
- Enlarged Sylvian fissures and basal cistern; and
- Narrowing of the sulci and subarachnoid spaces over the high convexity and midline surface of the brain.

Unlike the International Guidelines, periventricular changes are not considered essential in Japanese guidelines.

CSF Flow Void by MRI and CSF Flow Rate by Phase-contrast MRI

Cerebrospinal fluid flow void phenomenon over the cerebral aqueduct is considered to have a low diagnostic value. This lead to the development of cine MRI or phase-contrast MRI. The diagnostic sensitivity of CSF flow rate at the cerebral aqueduct using phase-contrast MRI is high.[15] But the diagnostic value has not been established.

Cine phase-contrast MRI helps in quantification of CSF flow in terms of stroke volume. Stroke volume is defined as the mean volume of CSF passing through the cerebral aqueduct in systole and diastole. Stroke volume greater than 42 μL may predict the likelihood of shunt responsiveness.[20] CSF stroke volume elevates after symptom onset, subsequently reaches a plateau after 18–20 months and then falls, implying that increased flow associated with ventriculomegaly might cause shear stress on periventricular tissues that would be reversible with shunting procedures.[21] Studies have also shown no correlation between outcome of a high-volume lumbar puncture or shunting and CSF stroke volume measured by phase-contrast MRI even at a median duration of 1 year.[22] What can be inferred from this is that there is insufficient evidence to establish phase-contrast MRI in prediction of response to shunt surgery, but increased CSF stroke volume is supportive for the diagnosis of NPH.

DIAGNOSTIC PROCEDURES

Five diagnostic studies can be used to assess patients who may have NPH.[23]

Routine Spinal Tap

In NPH routine CSF spinal tap may demonstrate normal CSF protein and glucose, and a white blood cell count of five or fewer cells per μL [or mm^3] and abnormal opening pressure of less than 200 mmH$_2$O. Absence of any of these should prompt alternate diagnosis. Diagnostic spinal tap may not be helpful in resolution of symptoms, but might help rule out alternate causes.[23]

Intermittent High-volume Tap

Symptoms and signs are first noted before the test. Approximately 30–60 mL of CSF is removed. Improvement of symptoms with careful removal of 30–60 mL of CSF may indicate an ensuing positive response to ventriculoperitoneal shunting.[24-26] Previous studies have shown that, patients who underwent high volume CSF Tap had a positive response to shunting at 3 months with 73% reporting benefit at 3 years.[26]

Prolonged Lumbar Drainage

Some studies have suggested 3–5 days of lumbar drainage via interval or constant pump-controlled removal of CSF combined with simultaneous assessment of the patient's symptoms to be more indicative of subsequent response to shunting procedures.[27,28] Two case series where 5–6 days of CSF diversion via lumbar drain proved 100% effective in predicting positive outcome to shunting.[27,28]

Intracranial Pressure

Evidence from intracranial monitoring devices over an extended period of time have shown intermittent spikes of elevated pressure. Demonstration of episodic waves of high pressure that are usually missed with routine lumbar puncture pressure measurements can be detected by placement of an intracranial pressure (ICP) monitor.[23]

Cerebrospinal Fluid Outflow Studies

Cerebrospinal fluid outflow studies help to determine the pressure response to outflow after infusion of a sterile solution at the rates of 0.5–5 mL/min.[23] A lumbar cistern access is established and sterile fluid is infuse. With the placement of a ventriculostomy tube, ICP is measured during the test and once after the release of CSF once the ICP has reached a certain level.[23] In some studies,[29,30] elevated outflow resistance helped in prediction of likely shunt-responsive patients. However a follow-up study of outcomes of 35 patients, the results were inconclusive.[30] Eventually, there is a lack of consensus about which diagnostic test predicts shunt responsiveness. Finally, there is no gold standard test to identify patients who will benefit from CSF diversion. These tests might ultimately help in the diagnosis of patients who likely have NPH.[23]

TREATMENT

Drug Treatment

There is no definitive drug therapy for INPH.[15] No evidence has been demonstrated regarding the benefits of anti-dementia and anti-Parkinson agents as symptomatic treatment.

Surgical intervention is the only treatment supported by high quality evidence. Although, some cases exhibit improvements in their symptoms with repeated CSF removal by lumbar puncture, there is no long-term effectiveness in cases where surgical intervention have proved efficacy.

Surgical Procedures

The surgical procedures for the treatment of INPH are the same as those for other types of communicating hydrocephalus. Those include: (i) Ventriculoperitoneal shunt; (ii) ventriculoatrial shunt and (iii) lumbo-peritoneal shunt. Another shunt of historical value is a ventriculoatrial shunt; was often performed on patients with INPH in the past. It is considered obsolete now.[15]

Ventriculoatrial Shunt

It is of historical value. It has been associated with lots of complications, including sepsis, endocarditis, cardiac wall perforation, cardiac tamponade, pleural effusion, kidney injury, pulmonary embolism, and pulmonary hypertension, which are very detrimental.[15]

Lumbo-peritoneal Shunt

Patients who show improvement in symptoms after a tap test, should be considered for a lumboperitoneal shunt, which is similar to the tap test and is not invasive to the brain (requiring penetration of a ventricle). Till date, there are no studies to demonstrate the superiority of lumboperitoneal shunt over other types of CSF shunts.[15] The advantages of a lumboperitoneal shunt over ventriculoperitoneal shunt is its lower risk of infections; however, shunt dysfunction is a common problem and spinal radiculopathy may be induced by displacement of the lumbar catheter, predominantly in older patients.[15]

Endoscopic Third Ventriculostomy

Few reports have shown improvement of symptoms following endoscopic third ventriculostomy, but imaging findings from individual cases are inconclusive. Endoscopic third ventriculostomy treatment is currently not considered to be beneficial for the treatment of INPH.[15]

Types of Shunt Systems

The shunt systems for INPH patients can be categorized by the following structural features:
- Adjustable or programmable valves
- Fixed differential pressure valves
- Gravity-assisted valve
- Flow-regulated valve
- Anti-siphon devices have been developed and administered to prevent excessive CSF

drainage, which can occur when the patient is in a sitting or standing position.

An anti-siphon device is either a supplementary device for the above valves or a built-in part.[15]

Adjustable or Programmable Valves

The pressure of the valve can be adjusted noninvasively even after installation. This is considered to be a major advantage because the NPH patients are generally noncompliant and readjustment of the pressures might be needed multiple times. Adjustable or programmable valves are presently recommended valves for INPH patients (recommendation grade B).[15]

Fixed Differential Pressure Valves

The flow of CSF is determined by a pressure gradient between the inlet and outlet of the valve. It is being considered widely because of its simple structure, low maintenance, stability of function and low cost. Based on the pressure gradient it creates, low (5–50 mmH$_2$O) or medium-pressure (51–110 mmH$_2$O) valves have been used for INPH patients. A low pressure valve is considered superior to a medium-pressure valve because of observed improvement rates of dementia and gait disturbance. However, medium- or high-pressure valves are now being preferred because of the low risk of over drainage, such as subdural effusion, as in the case of low-pressure valves. These valves are inferior to programmable valves because of its low effectiveness and high-probability of postoperative complications (recommendation grade C1).[15]

Gravity-assisted Valves

Gravity assisted valves are position-sensitive. Depending on whether the patient is supine or standing position these valves provides CSF flow path and resistance in two different ways. This valve is particularly useful in cases to prevent over drainage while standing. The direction of the valve is most important because it is not appropriate then it may not function. This valve is particularly useful in ventriculoperitoneal shunt.[15]

Flow-regulated Valves

The internal resistance varies automatically, according to the pressure on flow-regulated valves. When the pressure difference is settled, there is no flow across the valve. A major advantage of these types of valves is that there is no artifact on MRI.[15] However, there is no significant superiority or difference between this valve and differential pressure valves in terms of improvement rate, infection rate, failure rate of the shunt procedure, and the incidence of subdural effusion.[15]

Anti-siphon Devices

These anti-siphon devices can be used along with the CSF shunt systems A–D described above, whenever there is excessive flow, when the patient is in a sitting or standing position. These devices are either built into the valves A through D or used with them as auxiliary/supplementary devices.

COMPLICATIONS

Postoperative complications include shunt infection, shunt failure, headache, meningoencephalitis, and subdural hygroma/hematoma due to CSF over drainage.

OUTCOME

Outcomes of surgery at 3 years and 5 years have been reported. The efficacy of shunt procedures maintained for the short-term ranged from 3 to 6 months in 64–96% of patients and at 1 year in 41–95%.[15] The efficacy of shunt procedures maintained for the long term ranged from 3 to 5 years in 28–91% of patients.[15] The best improvement rate was observed for gait disturbance, between 58 and 90%.[15] Dementia symptoms improved in 29–80% of patients.[15] Urinary incontinence symptoms improved in 20–82.5% of patients.[15,31]

REFERENCES

1. Gleason PL, Black PM, Matsumae M. The neurobiology of normal pressure hydrocephalus. Neurosurg Clin North Am. 1993;4:667-75.
2. Vanneste JA. Diagnosis and management of normal pressure hydrocephalus. J Neurol 2000;247:5-14.

3. Vanneste JA, Augustijn P, Dirven C, et al. Shunting normal-pressure hydrocephalus: Do the benefits outweigh the risks? A multicenter study and literature review. Neurology 1992;42:54-9.
4. Akai K, Uchigasaki S, Tanaka U, et al. Normal pressure hydrocephalus. Neuropathological study. Acta Pathol Jpn. 1987;37:97-110.
5. Kudo T, Mima T, Hashimoto R, et al. Tau protein is a potential biological marker for normal pressure hydrocephalus. Psychiatry Clin Neurosci. 2000;54: 199-202.
6. Kondziella D, Sonnewald U, Tullberg M, et al. Brain metabolism in adult chronic hydrocephalus. J Neurochem. 2008;106:1515-24.
7. Larsson A, Stephensen H, Wikkelsö C. Normal pressure hydrocephalus. Demonstration status improved by shunt surgery. Läkartidningen 1995;92:545-50
8. Mori E. Gait disturbance in idiopathic normal pressure hydrocephalus. Brain Nerve. 2008;60:219-224.
9. Estañol BV. Gait apraxia in communicating hydrocephalus. J Neurol Neurosurg Psychiatry. 1981;44:305-18.
10. Knutsson E, Lying-Tunnel U. Gait apraxia in normal-pressure hydrocephalus: Patterns of movement and muscle activation. Neurology. 1985;35:155-60.
11. Lindqvist G, Andersson H, Bilting M, et al. Normal pressure hydrocephalus: psychiatric findings before and after shunt operation classified in a new diagnostic system for organic psychiatry. Acta Psychiatr Scand. 1993;88(Suppl 373):18-32.
12. Tullberg M, Hellström P, Piechnik SK, et al. Impaired wakefulness is associated with reduced anterior cingulated CBF in patients with normal pressure hydrocephalus. Acta Neurol Scand. 2004;110:322-30.
13. Ahlberg J, Norlén L, Blomstrand C, et al. Outcome of shunt operation on urinary incontinence in normal pressure hydrocephalus predicted by lumbar puncture. J Neurol Neurosurg Psychiatry. 1988;51:105-8.
14. Sakakibara R, Kanda T, Sekido T, et al. Mechanism of bladder dysfunction in idiopathic normal pressure hydrocephalus. Neurourol Urodyn. 2008;27:507-10
15. Mori E, Ishikawa M, Kato T, et al. Japanese Society of Normal Pressure Hydrocephalus. Neurol Med Chir (Tokyo). 2012;52(11):775-809.
16. Miyake H, Kajimoto Y, Tsuji M, et al. Development of a quick reference table for setting programmable pressure valves in patients with idiopathic normal pressure hydrocephalus. Neurol Med Chir (Tokyo). 2008;48:427-32.
17. Shirane R, Hayashi T, Miyake H, et al. Cerebrospinal fluid shunt devices: An historical perspective. No Shinkei Geka Journal. 2010;19:510-7.
18. Lavinio A, Harding S, Van Der Boogaard F, et al. Magnetic field interactions in adjustable hydrocephalus shunts. J Neurosurg Pediatr. 2008;2:222-8.
19. Damasceno BP. Neuroimaging in normal pressure hydrocephalus. Dementia & Neuropsychologia. 2015;9(4):350-5.
20. Bradley WG Jr, Scalzo D, Queralt J, et al. Normal-pressure hydrocephalus: Evaluation with cerebrospinal fluid flow measurements at MR imaging. Radiology. 1996;198:523-9.
21. Scollato A, Tenenbaum R, Bahl G, et al. Changes in aqueductal CSF stroke volume and progression of symptoms in patients with unshunted idiopathic normal pressure hydrocephalus. AJNR Am J Neuroradiol. 2008;29:192-7.
22. Kahlon B, Annertz M, Stahlberg F, et al. Is aqueductal stroke volume, measured with cine phase contrast magnetic resonance imaging scans useful in predicting outcome of shunt surgery in suspected normal pressure hydrocephalus? Neurosurgery. 2007;60:124-9.
23. Verrees M, Selman WR. Management of normal pressure hydrocephalus. Am Fam Physician. 2004;70(6): 1071-8.
24. Gleason PL, Black PM, Matsumae M. The neurobiology of normal pressure hydrocephalus. Neurosurg Clin North Am. 1993;4:667-75.
25. Meier U, Zeilinger FS, Kintzel D. Signs, symptoms and course of normal pressure hydrocephalus in comparison with cerebral atrophy. Acta Neurochir (Wien) 1999;141:1039-48.
26. Mori K. Management of idiopathic normal-pressure hydrocephalus: A multiinstitutional study conducted in Japan. J Neurosurg. 2001;95:970-3.
27. Chen IH, Huang CI, Liu HC, et al. Effectiveness of shunting in patients with normal pressure hydrocephalus predicted by temporary, controlled-resistance, continuous lumbar drainage: A pilot study. J Neurol Neurosurg Psychiatry. 1994;57:1430-2.
28. Haan J, Thomeer RT. Predictive value of temporary external lumbar drainage in normal pressure hydrocephalus. Neurosurgery. 1988;22:388-91.
29. Boon AJ, Tans JT, Delwel EJ, et al. The Dutch normal-pressure hydrocephalus study. How to select patients for shunting? An analysis of four diagnostic criteria. Surg Neurol 2000;53:201-7.
30. Meier U, Bartels P. The importance of the intrathecal infusion test in the diagnostic of normal-pressure hydrocephalus. Eur Neurol. 2001;46:178-86.
31. Hebb AO, Cusimano MD. Idiopathic normal pressure hydrocephalus: A systematic review of diagnosis and outcome. Neurosurgery. 2001;49:1166-84.

CHAPTER 6

Nonmotor Rehabilitation in Stroke

Philo H Philomin, Bhanu Kesavamurthy

INTRODUCTION

Stroke is an important cause of chronic disability worldwide. It leads to persistent neurobehavioral, language, cognitive, perceptional, and functional deficits amongst stroke survivors. Cognitive impairment is noted in 35% of patients 3 months following stroke and around 32% of patients up to 3 years following the onset of their first stroke.[1] There are multiple interventions that treat cognitive impairment and language disabilities following a stroke, and in turn improves the person's ability to perform functional activities. At the turn of the millennium, multiple factors such as increased understanding of the neuronal plasticity and the effects of electrical stimulation on motor evoked potentials led to the revival of interests in the various brain stimulation techniques for rehabilitation.[2] Intensive cognitive rehabilitation approaches targeting attention, information processing speed, executive function, and memory have been shown to have positive effects on the cognitive deficits.

PROCESSES IN CEREBRAL RECOVERY AFTER STROKE (FLOWCHART 1)

Recovery of function following stroke depends on either restoration or compensatory reorganization of the damaged neural/computational modules supporting particular cognitive domains.[3]

Cognitive impairment is a major sequel after an ischemic stroke, even in patients with good functional recovery. The compromise in different cognitive domains predicts the future functional disability. Cognition and perception are a dynamic process which constantly changes and reacts to both internal and external

- Restitution – Restoring the functionality of damaged neural tissue

- Sustituition – Reorganization of partly spared neural pathways to relearn lost functions

- Compensation – Improvement of the disparity between the impaired skills of a patient and the demands of their environment

FLOWCHART 1: Process in cerebral recovery after stroke.

stimuli. Cognitive and perceptual (processing) dysfunction can severely impair a person's ability to participate in routine daily activities. Therapists must address neurobehavioral impairments according to the situation and can be modified to the person's needs and goals. Hence, a general approach might not work in all patients and it has to be planned for individual patient needs. Cognitive rehabilitation is a "systematic, functionally oriented service of therapeutic activities that is based on assessment and understanding of the patient's brain-behavioral deficits".[4] Neuroenhancement is the use of neuroscience based techniques to enhance cognitive function by acting directly on the human brain and nervous system, thus, altering its properties to increase the performance.[2]

APPROACH TO PERCEPTUAL AND COGNITIVE IMPAIRMENT

The perceptual and cognitive impairments are treated by two approaches: (i) the functional/adaptive approach; (ii) the remediation/restoration approach. A combined approach during stroke rehabilitation is more effective.[5]

The Functional/Adaptive Approach

The patient tries adapting to the deficits, by changing the environmental parameters of a task to facilitate function. Uses the person's strengths to compensate for loss of function.[5] Practicing functional activities based on what the person receiving therapy wants to do, needs to do, or has to do in an environment.

Environmental adaptations (i.e., keeping the required grooming items on the right side of the sink in a person with neglect, using contrasting colors for a plate and doormat for a patient with figure-ground difficulties. Creating a routine and constant atmosphere with repeated performance in familiar activities is a successful strategy for these patients).

Compensatory strategy training approaches (i.e., scanning strategy such as the "Lighthouse Strategy" to improve attention to the left side of the environment for those living with neglect.

For those with memory impairment an alarm clock can be to remind them to take a medicines at a particular time).

Remediation, Restoration/Transfer of Training Approach

Use of techniques to improve the actual cognitive or perceptual skills affected by the stroke. Uses deficit-specific cognitive and perceptual retraining activities depending on the pattern of impairment. Examples of interventions: cognitive and perceptual table-top "exercises", parquetry blocks, specialized computer software programs, cancellation tasks, block designs, pegboard design copying, puzzles, sequencing cards, gesture imitation, picture matching, design copying.

In patients with impaired learning potential and awareness, a domain-specific training would help. In domain-specific training a specific activity is performed repetitively using vanishing cues, in which cues are given at every step of task and are later gradually removed. The goal is to establish a program in which the patient can successfully perform the task with a minimum number of cues. This type of training is hyperspecific, and the learning associated with it persists only if the task and environmental characteristics remain unchanged. It is proposed that an integrated treatment strategy comprising of all the approaches simultaneously would be beneficial.[5]

INTERVENTIONS FOR SENSORY, VISUOSPATIAL, AND PERCEPTUAL DEFICITS (BOX 1)

Perceptual performance is "the ability to organize, process and interpret incoming visual information, tactile-kinesthetic information, or both, and to act appropriately on the basis of the information received".[6] Somatosensory impairment for multiple modalities is noted after a stroke and correlates with the stroke severity. The incidence of visual neglect varies and they range from 13 to 85%. Neglect specific therapeutic approaches includes structured

> **Box 1: Interventions for visuospatial and perceptual deficits**
>
> - Compensatory interventions: Saccadic eye movement training, training in visual search strategies, training eye movements for reading, use of eye blinks or color cues, training in activities of daily living
> - Substitutive interventions: Prisms eye patches, adapted lighting, magnification, environmental modification

therapy sessions, computerized therapy and prescription of aids, but their use has not been shown to impact long term on disability or independence. The use of compensatory scanning, visual restitution training (restitutive intervention) or prisms (substitutive intervention) for patients helps in improving the visual field deficits.[7,8] The scanning training is where the subject is asked to scan the environment while being mobile and static with rotational activities. The light house strategy is where the subject is to pay clear attention to the right and left while the therapists shows the correct degree and pace of head turning using a light house model.[9]

Use of tools like cane, walker can extend extrapersonal visual space in patients with neglect, it improves perceptual-motor performance and becomes an effective rehabilitation aid. Rehabilitation for many perceptual deficits post-stroke includes functional training, sensory stimulation, strategy training and task repetition. The transfer of training approach assumes that practice on a particular perceptual task will improve performance on similar perceptual tasks. The functional approach strives to promote functional independence through the repetitive practice of particular tasks, usually activities of daily living (ADL). Transfer of strategies from trained tasks to nontrained (related) tasks is very important in terms of the clinical success of a therapy program. In strategy training, the occurrence of transfer is expected as the training program is not aimed at relearning specific tasks, but at teaching patients new ways to handle the problems resulting from the impairment. Thermal intervention and electrical stimulation are found effective in improving upper limb sensation and function.

FUNCTIONAL MEMORY

Memory strategy training includes training by internalized mnemonic strategies, behavioral strategies (e.g., placing keys in the same place routinely), and external compensatory strategies and tools (e.g., using to-do lists like memory notebook).

Errorless learning: The learning process is structured by the therapist to avoid errors and in the trial-and-error learning we can encourage guessing. Errorless learning activates the implicit memory systems and improves the performance without the patient awareness. Targeting interventions like vigilance training for vigilance deficits and selective attention training can be done when multiple domains of attention are affected. Attention process training with pharmacotherapy or psychotherapy have shown complementary effects, with improvements noted in working and other memory skills, as well as in executive control. Metacognitive strategy training enhances that self-monitoring and self-regulation (e.g., remembering safety instructions when using a walker) is required to live independently in patients with executive dysfunction post-stroke.[10]

Cognitive training: It is a therapeutic method which is aimed at preventing cognitive decline and promotes neuroplasticity. Cognitive training can delay the cognitive decline by slowing the progression of the neurobiological changes that contribute to memory impairment (Flowchart 2).

ATTENTION DEFICITS

Attention is "the voluntary control over more automatic brain systems, and be able to select and manipulate sensory and stored information briefly or for sustained periods of time". The difficulty to attend to a task can be taken as a lack of motivation or neglect. Before planning appropriate treatment goals, the accurate

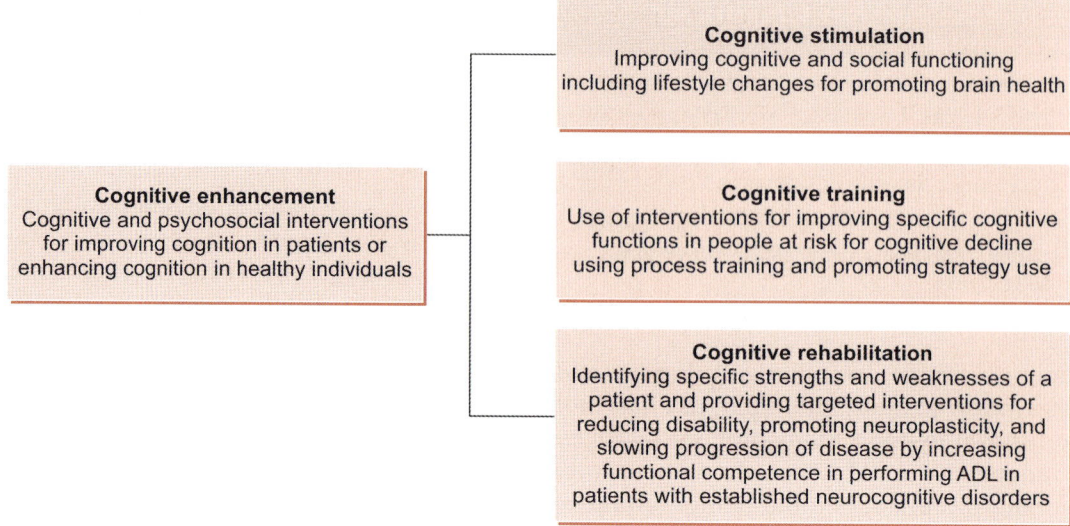

ADL, activities of daily living.

FLOWCHART 2: Memory training strategies.

assessment of the attention is required. The goal is to couple the patient's attention with the result required, the instructions to the patient should be in the logical sequence of the order in which the steps are to be executed and should allow the patient to attend to each step. Patient is required to pause in between, as it gives enough time to shift focus and process the information. Systematic training approach with a series of tasks with progressively increasing attentional demands results in memory improvement and task attention.[5]

Attention Deficits: Strategies for Clinicians and Caretakers[5]

- Avoiding clutter, visual distracters, and distracting environments while performing tasks
- Maintaining an organized and uncluttered manner of filling systems, by labeling cupboards and cabinets. Daily checklists for work and routine ADL
- Learning strategies for self-instruction, self-pacing and time pressure management. In time pressure management patients are taught compensatory cognitive strategies, when in time pressured situations. They can prior rehearse the tasks and also modify the task environment when required
- Learning to manage the effort and emotional responses themselves during a task
- Learning to monitor and to share the attentional resources while multitasking
- To avoid distraction at home due to auditory and visual stimuli, can wear ear plugs, keep radios and phones off, close doors and curtains.

APRAXIA TRAINING

Strategy Training

Patients are taught strategies to compensate for the presence of apraxia. Interventions were focused on errors related to:

- *Initiation*: Developing a plan of action and selection of required and correct objects
- *Execution*: Performance of the plan
- *Control*: Controlling and correcting the activity for an adequate result.[5]

Errorless Completion and Training of Details

Errorless learning or completion is a technique in which the person does the activity and learns from it. Incase error occurs the therapist helps to correct them. Specific interventions included:

- Guiding the hand through a difficult aspect of the task
- Perform the same task simultaneously with the patient being besides him (parallel position)
- Asking the patient to copy the task demonstrated by the therapist after a while.[5]

Exploration Training

Exploration training focused on directing the patient's attention to the structure of an object and solve mechanical problems embedded in tasks (i.e., prongs on a fork, serrations on a butter knife, bristles on a toothbrush).[5,11]

Interventions for Functional Limitations due to Apraxia[5,11]

- Using functional task specific approach for each individuals
- "Tap into" the subjects daily routines and habits
- Client-centered/context specific approach—both the caregiver and the patient are to choose the main task to focus on at the appropriate time and environment of the day
- Using strategy training interventions to develop internal or external compensations for routine functional activities
- Error-specific interventions
- Practice functional activities with vanishing cues
- Providing graded assistance by instructions, assistance, or feedback during task performance.

AGNOSIA TRAINING[5,11]

Visual Agnosia

- Compensating using other senses like tactile sensation, which helps recognizing figures and shapes using the kinesthetic sense. The other modalities are the auditory and olfactory senses
- Make them aware of the deficits or else they might underestimate the consequences and to explain the visual features of objects before telling the name
- Using the spatial and location clues to identify objects and people (e.g., organizing a room so that required objects are assigned to a particular spatial locations such as school clothes on the right side of the dresser and casual clothes on the left, having a sofa as a landmark to find route)
- A piecemeal reconstruction method using feature-by-feature analysis. Teaching importance of verbal memory skills and verbal reasoning to analyze the piecemeal visual information into a complete picture (e.g., "it's a person, no it's a dress, it's short, and it must be a shirt")
- Usage of color clues, labels on objects (e.g., Velcro on the phone receiver or yellow tape on lock)
- Can strategize activities watching other people (e.g., in case of difficulty in finding the utensils during a meal, can learn to find the items by watching others at the meal)
- Learning to identify real objects by focusing on the surface texture, colors and depth cues, as they are more easily identified than drawings or pictures.

Prosopagnosia

- Characteristics of the gait (e.g., speed, hand movements, noise from shoes) and voice recognition can help identifying people
- Using the localization clues as to who sits next to me at work and who sits on my left at work
- Characteristic features of a person like an eye color, a scar to be remembered.

Topographic Disorientation

Learn to navigation in the house by routinely starting at the same point in the house. Using the kinesthetic (e.g., number of steps and turns taken to reach), vestibular cues and visual cues like marking different colors in the key rooms of the house from the past memories to help learn the directions to navigate around.

Tactile Agnosia/Astereognosis

Combination of both tactile and visual stimuli (e.g., recognizing two-dimensional and three-dimensional objects).

Alexia

It can be intervened by teaching to read the letters by tracing from palm of the hand.

Pure Word Deafness

Teach use of contextual cues, intonation, gestures, and facial expressions.

NEUROENHANCEMENT

Neuroenhancement tools work directly on our nervous systems to improve our cognitive function and increase our capabilities (Box 2). Neuroenhancement by noninvasive stimulation brain stimulation has received much attention and has made great progress in recent times.[2] Studying the effect of multimodal neuroenhancement on brain connectivity by cognitive training, neurofeedback, and brain stimulation methods is more powerful than the use of single methods alone. Recent advances in novel brain computer interface technologies promises to provide assistance in neurological disorders.

> **Box 2: Neuroenhancement methods of neurorehabilitation**
>
> - Brain stimulation techniques
>   - Transcranial direct current stimulation (tDCS)
>   - Transcranial alternating current stimulation (tACS)
>   - Transcranial random noise stimulation (tRNS)
>   - Transcranial magnetic stimulation (TMS)
>   - Deep brain stimulation (DBS)
> - Neurofeedback
>   - EEG neurofeedback
>   - Functional MRI neurofeedback
>   - EEG-fMRI neurofeedback
> - Cognitive training
>
> EEG, electroencephalography; fMRI, functional magnetic resonance imaging; MRI, magnetic resonance imaging.

NEUROFEEDBACK

Neurofeedback is a method of noninvasive modulation of brain activity which is used in treating neurological disorders as well as for enhancing cognitive performance of the brain.[12] Neurofeedback uses neuroimaging techniques like functional magnetic resonance imaging (fMRI) and electroencephalography to obtain real-time measures of activity in the brain, thus enabling self-regulation of brain function by the individual. The fMRI is also helpful in assessing recovery in patients with post-stroke aphasia.

SPEECH AND LANGUAGE

Aphasia is a common neuropsychological effect seen in about one third of all left hemispheric strokes in acute phase. Post-stroke aphasia can be managed in the early phase by intensive delivery of information processing tasks, restorative and compensatory aphasia treatment strategies. Intensive treatment for aphasia rehabilitation through constraint-induced language/aphasia therapy (CILT/CIAT) improves outcomes. The CILT is a method where efficacy of the treatment can be improved by constraining compensatory strategies of communication like gesturing, drawing, writing and elliptical speech.[3] Approach to speech rehabilitation is given in box 3.

Stimulation of the lesional or contralesional regions of the brain by noninvasive brain stimulation procedures help in aphasia as intra- and interhemispheric interactions are involved in language recovery. The repetitive transcranial magnetic stimulation (rTMS) is utilized as a complementary treatment approach in nonfluent aphasia by inhibiting the areas of the language network which are abnormally activated. Suppression of activation in the right homotopic frontal speech areas using 1Hz rTMS has a modulating effect on the other neural networks for language. The cognitive domains like picture word verification speeds up on stimulating the Broca's area and the picture naming on stimulating Wernicke's area. Transcranial direct current stimulation (tDCS)

> **Box 3: Approach to speech rehabilitation[13]**
> - Stimulation: Facilitation approach
> - Modality model approach
> - Processing approach
> - Nondominant hemispheric approach
> - Linguistic approach
> - Functional communication approach
> - Life participation approach
> - Biological approach

and rTMS have resulted in improvement in the receptive and explorative modalities of language and offers future supplementary approaches to conventional therapy. The widespread use of neuroimaging in future research will help us understand better about language recovery in stroke.

FATIGUE AND MOOD DISORDERS

The prevalence of PSD has ranged from 5 to 63% and it peaks three to six months after a stroke. Post-stroke fatigue and mood disorders can be distressing and it impacts negatively on the rehabilitation. As fatigue after stroke may have several causative factors, there are a number of potential interventions, including psychological (counseling, cognitive behavior therapy) or physical treatment (graded exercise).[3]

Psychotherapy along with pharmacotherapy helps in improving mood and prevents depression. Cognitive and graded activity training (COGRAT) is a treatment approach which helps in improving post-stroke fatigue by changing cognitions and enhancing physical fitness by graded activity programs in small groups over 12 weeks. The activities in the programs include walking on a treadmill, strength training, and homework assignments.

CONCLUSION

Stroke-related disability has a great impact on the patient's quality of life to live independently, and an effective neurorehabilitation will help in the recovery. As the rates of stroke increasing, it is important that we continue to foster innovation in stroke rehabilitation. Till date only a selective set of cognitive domains are effectively addressed in cognitive rehabilitation and we frequently fails to address long-term outcomes and generalization of treatments to typical daily activities. More research is required into the correct assessment of certain features of visual perceptual disorders to help improve future methods for rehabilitation.

Still, a wide gap persists between investigational treatments and our evolving theories of brain function. The underdevelopment of the rehabilitation settings could be due to the challenges presented by individual differences and we are still not sure of many of these interventions on functional recovery. With further research on noninvasive brain stimulation techniques their potential usefulness in the real world will emerge over time. These new techniques offer great hope for the future of stroke rehabilitation. Research in the area of neuro-rehabilitative methods of neuroenhancement will continue, and along with other measures may spark a new age in the way we think about treating neurocognitive dysfunction.

REFERENCES

1. Tatemichi T, Desmond D, Stern Y, et al. Cognitive impairment after stroke: frequency, patterns, and relationship to functional abilities. J Neurol Neurosurg Psychiatry. 1994;57(2):202-7.
2. Vincent P. Clark A, Parasuraman R. Neuroenhancement: Enhancing brain and mind in health and in disease. Neuro Image. 2014;85:889-94.
3. Brewer L, Horgan F, Hickey A, et al. Stroke rehabilitation: Recent advances and future therapies J Med. 2013;106:11-25.
4. Cicerone KD, Dahlberg C, Malec JF, et al. Evidence-based cognitive rehabilitation: Updated review of the literature from 1998 through 2002. Arch Phys Med Rehabil. 2005;86:1681-92.
5. Gillen G, Rubio KB. Treatment of cognitive-perceptual deficits: A Function-Based Approach . Stroke rehabilitation book 4th edition; 2016.
6. Jutai JW, Bhogal SK, Foley NC, et al. Treatment of visual perceptual disorders post stroke. Stroke Rehabil. 2003;10(2):77-106.
7. Ackroyd K, Riddoch MJ, Humphreys GW, et al. Widening the sphere of influence: Using a tool to extend extrapersonal visual space in a patient with severe neglect. Neurocase. 2002;8:1-12.

8. Pollock A, Hazelton C, Henderson CA, et al. Interventions for visual field defects in patients with stroke. Cochrane Database Syst Rev. 2011;(10):CD008388.
9. Neimer, Janet P. Visual imagery training for patients with visual perceptual deficits following right hemisphere cerebrovascular accidents: A case presenting the light house strategy. Rehabilitation Psychology. 2002;47(4):426-37.
10. Shigak CL, Fre SH, Barrett AM. Rehabilitation of post stroke cognition. Semin Neurol. 2014;34(5):496-503.
11. Gillen G. Cognitive and perceptual rehabilitation: Optimizing function, St. Louis, 2009, Mosby/Elsevier.
12. Zotev V, Phillips R, Yuan H, et al. Self-regulation of human brain activity using simultaneous real-time fMRI and EEG neurofeedback. Neuroimage. 2014;85 Pt 3:985-95.
13. Horners J, Loverso FL, Rothi. Models of aphasia treatment. In: Chapey R (Ed). Language intervention strategies in adult aphasia. 3rd ed. Baltimore: Williams Wilkins;1994. P.135-45.

CHAPTER 7

Sleep Disorders in Parkinson's Disease: From Research to Clinical Practice

Vinoth K Selvaraj

INTRODUCTION

Sleep disorders are very common in Parkinson's disease (PD). Sleep disorders comes under the "nonmotor components" of PD and it can predate its motor manifestations. Patients may complain of difficulty in initiating sleep, fragmented sleep due to frequent awakenings in the night, early morning awakenings, inadequate night sleep followed by excessive daytime sleepiness (EDS), snoring, nightmares, hallucinations, vivid dreams, confusion arousals, panic attacks, periodic limb movements (PLMs), restless legs syndrome (RLS), rapid eye movement (REM) sleep behavioral disorder (RBD) etc.

The sleep disturbance in PD is explained by:[1]
- Primary involvement of sleep regulating structures
- Secondary involvement through motor, depressive and dysautonomic symptoms
- Tertiary involvement through pharmacologic measures.

Primary Involvement of Sleep Regulating Structures

Various anatomic structures are involved in the generation and maintenance of the sleep-wake cycle in human beings. The cortex, brainstem, thalamus, hypothalamus, limbic system, basal ganglia are the structures involved in the generation of sleep. The substrates being pedunculopontine nucleus, lateral dorsal tegmentum, dorsal midbrain raphe nucleus, locus ceruleus, tuberomammillary nucleus of hypothalamus, periaqueductal gray matter of midbrain etc. They undergo degeneration resulting in sleep disturbance. Many neurotransmitters like glutamate, γ-aminobutyric acid, glycine, hypocretin/orexin, melanin-concentrating hormone, melatonin, histamine, acetylcholine, dopamine, serotonin, and noradrenaline are implicated in the regulation of sleep. The degenerative process may actually begin at a very early stage in some patients and at a later stage in others.[2]

Secondary Involvement through Motor, Depressive, and Dysautonomic Symptoms

Rigidity, tremor and bradykinesia, are the cardinal features of PD. These symptoms recur at night, during the lighter stages of sleep resulting in nocturnal akinesia which gives rise to discomfort and sleep disturbance. Patients are also forced to sleep for long periods in the same posture, causing sensory disturbance like numbness and pain. Muscle cramps also causes sleep disturbance. Periodic limb movements are more common in PD even in early untreated patients.

Tremor may be present for 30% of time spent in bed causing nocturnal wakefulness. It disappears in REM sleep and present with reduced amplitude in nonrapid eye movement (NREM) sleep. Rigidity and cogwheeling are also reduced but present during sleep. Sleep related respiratory muscle dysfunction is due to abnormal tone in upper airway muscles, incoordination of respiratory muscles, and fluctuations in muscle functioning. The immediate sensation on awakening is a sensation of suffocation interpreted as sleep apnea.[3] Parkinson's disease patients with severe sleep disturbance and excessive day time sleepiness have irregular sleep-wake pattern. As there is alteration in the circadian regulation in PD patients there is a change in the functioning of autonomic nervous system.[4] Insomnia reported in 32% of the PD patients.[4] The most common complaints by the patients are defect in the sleep initiation, sleep fragmentation and early awakenings. The prevalence of insomnia increases with age.

Depression is the common cause of sleep disturbance in elderly. There is difficulty in falling asleep and remaining asleep. Early morning awakening is a cardinal feature seen in depression. Insomnia is the earliest sign of mood disturbance and it occurs before the clinical evidence of depression. Forty percent of the PD patients have depression.[5] The causes of depression ranges from neurochemical imbalances associated with PD to the consequences of living with the chronic progressive degenerative illness. There is no correlation of the depression with age, disease duration, severity, and cognitive impairment.

Psychosis affects one-fifth of the PD patients[6] and causes sleep problems. Frequency of psychosis increases with age and it also correlates with cognitive impairment. Hallucinations can occur in any stage of PD either spontaneously or secondary to medications. Up to 40% of PD patients having hallucinations are associated with RBD.[6] Around 50% of the PD patients complains of pain due to foot dyskinesia which is related to the off state or insufficient dose of dopaminergic therapy.[7] Adjustment of the dosages and analgesics provide relief. The prevalence of cognitive impairment rises with age. In a cohort study[8] more than three quarters of the patients developed dementia during a 8-year study period. Early hallucinations and akinetic rigid phenotype are associated with increased risk of dementia. Autonomic disturbances are common in PD.[9] Dysphagia, paroxysmal sweating are specific to PD. Nocturia, day time urge incontinence, constipation, impotence, hypothermia are related to the aging process or may be secondary to antiparkinsonian medications. Nocturia is the commonest symptom encountered in clinical practice. There is increase in prevalence of nocturia in PD. Eighty percent of the PD patients have two or more episodes of nocturia per month and 33% urinate more than three times per night.[10] The frequency of nocturia correlates with the disease severity. There is an increase in urinary frequency when the dopaminergic medication wears off. So a long acting medication given at the night will be helpful. Other autonomic features like night time blood pressure variability or paradoxical hypertension occur at later stage of the disease.

Tertiary Involvement through Pharmacologic Treatment

Pharmacological treatment influence the sleep in different ways, depending on the drug and its administration schedule. Antiparkinsonian medications can both aggravate and relieve nocturnal symptoms. Levodopa (L-dopa) plays a dual role. Low doses of L-dopa have a sedating, sleep-enhancing effect, whereas higher doses have a stimulating, sleep-inhibiting effect. Respiration may be initially enhanced by central L-dopa stimulation and later inhibited by peripheral action of L-dopa on chemoreceptor reflexes. Levodopa may also results in night time hallucinations. Levodopa may relieve night time akinesia and reduce the muscle tone in PD patients. As the L-dopa wears off in the early morning hours, akinetic episodes occurs resultig in early morning awakenings. Nightmares are reported in 32% of PD patients.[10] There is a positive correlation of the nightmares with the staging, severity, and L-dopa dosage. Reducing the dose of dopaminergic medications and the anticholinergic agents helps to relieve the symptoms.

SYMPTOMS OF SLEEP DISTURBANCES IN PARKINSON'S DISEASE

Insomnia

Sleep maintenance insomnia is very common than sleep initiation insomnia. In this form of insomnia, the patient wakes after 2–3 hours feeling relatively refreshed and is unable to fall back to consolidated sleep. The sleep remains fragmented throughout the night. In the daytime, sleepiness recurs and the patient takes multiple short naps. Although sleep is not consolidated, the total quantity of sleep over a 24-hour period is normal. Secondary factors may contribute including decreased body movements, nocturia, pain, anxiety, depression, and vivid dreams.

Hypersomnia

Excessive daytime sleepiness is defined as symptomatic daytime somnolence with frequent sleep periods. Pramipexole, nonergot dopamine agonist have caused drowsiness and sudden irresistible naps. These attacks were reduced after the discontinuation of the drug. Daytime sleepiness correlated better with first occurrence of autonomic failure, longer duration or advanced stage of the disease, advanced age of the patient, and male sex.

Parasomnia

The most common parasomnia is the RBD. Rapid eye movement sleep behavior disorder is characterized by loss of REM sleep related hypotonia associated with abnormal motor activities and the patients may enact the dreams in REM sleep causing injury to themselves or to the bed partners. Rapid eye movement sleep behavior disorder may be primary or secondary, most of them are due to neurodegenerative diseases like PD, multiple system atrophy, corticobasal degeneration, dementia with Lewy bodies, olivopontocerebellar atrophy, and progressive supranuclear palsy. The prevalence of REM disorder varies from 15 to 47%.[11] Rapid eye movement sleep behavior disorder predates the motor symptoms in PD in 52 % of individuals.[11]

Rapid eye movement sleep behavior disorder is common in akinetic-rigid phenotype of PD, and it is associated with high frequency of falls, less responsive to dopaminergic medications than PD patients without RBD and PD patients with RBD have high incidence of cognitive impairment, impaired color discrimination, diminished olfaction, dysautonomia, increased prevalence of sleep walking behavior. Increased muscle activity in REM sleep, which is an early sign of RBD is reported in asymptomatic patients who have PD.[11] Individuals with RBD have significantly increased risk of developing Parkinsonism if there is decreased nigrosriatal dopaminergic activity in the functional imaging over the next decade.

CONTRIBUTION OF MOTOR DYSFUNCTION TO SLEEP DISTURBANCE IN PARKINSON'S DISEASE

Motor disorders that appear at night in PD include tremor, rigidity, bradykinesia, painful dystonia, dyskinesias, PLMs, restless legs, akathisia, RBD.

Role of Tremor

Electromyography recording of the muscles involved in tremor during wakefulness shows rhythmic repetitive muscle contractions during the NREM sleep. The repetitive muscle contraction is considered the equivalent of Parkinsonian tremor during sleep which contributes to light and fragmented sleep.

Role of Rigidity

Although muscle tone decreases during the different stages of sleep, variable degrees of rigidity can persist in Parkinsonian patients during the night, especially those who have motor fluctuations. This rigidity accounts for stiffness, mainly of axial distribution, and is a major contributor to nocturnal pain in PD. This is responsible for poor nocturnal mobility that manifest as impairment in making postural adjustments like difficulty turning over in bed. Painful dystonia occur in the early morning, but dystonic spasms and postures, usually localized to the legs, can appear at any time during the night. The pathophysiology of nocturnal painful dystonia is similar to that of the off-period dystonia experienced by patients with motor fluctuation during the day. Levodopa-induced dyskinesias are more intense in the evening, due to cumulative effect of the recent L-dopa doses. The alerting effect of L-dopa cause delayed onset of sleep. When the patient arouse from sleep at night the dyskinesias reappear and prevents the patient from going back to sleep. Nighttime motor manifestations is related to the deficit in the dopaminergic tone during the night as it well responds to the controlled release formulations of L-dopa.

RESTLESS LEGS SYNDROME

It is the most common movement disorder, not commonly recognized. The patients has an unpleasant, uncomfortable sensations in the legs predominantly in the evening or night hours which causes an intense urge to move the legs and the movements like stretching, walking relieves the unpleasant sensations partially or completely. It may associated with a positive family history, presence of PLMs in sleep or wakefulness and response to dopamine. Eighty percent of the RLS patients have PLMs. Restless legs syndrome mainly causes difficulty in sleep initiation. Recent hypothesis states that reduced dopamine cellular function secondary to local iron deficiency is the pathophysiology behind RLS. Iron is an essential cofactor for tyrosine hydroxylase, the rate-limiting enzyme involved in dopamine synthesis, and iron deficiency decreases the number of dopamine D2 receptor binding sites, so the current research focus is centered on iron-dopamine dysfunction. Studies shows the site of central nervous system involvement in RLS is the brain stem, but the spinal cord may be one of the probable site. This disorder increases in prevalence with age and it is seen in 15% of the elderly patients. This movement causes frequent awakenings and arousals, thereby disrupting the sleep. Total 20.8% of the PD patients have RLS, which is twice that of the control population.[12]

PERIODIC LIMB MOVEMENTS IN SLEEP

Periodic limb movements are stereotyped limb movements, present in the REM sleep characterized by dorsiflexion movements of the ankle and flexion movements of the knee and hip for a period of 0.5–10 seconds with an average interval of 20–40 seconds and at least four consecutive movements should be present.

Periodic limb movements is seen in at least 80% of patients with RLS. Periodic limb movements occurs most commonly in RLS but may also occur in a large number of other medical, neurological, and sleep disorders and with medications like (e.g., selective serotonin reuptake inhibitors, tricyclic antidepressants) and even in normal individuals, particularly in those older than 65 years. There is also a growing body of evidence that PLMS may simply be a polysomnography observation and does not have any clinical significance.

Polysomnography Findings in Parkinson's Disease

Patients with PD have decreased total sleep time and frequent awakenings. Stage 2 NREM sleep show reduction in the sleep spindles and K complexes. Slow-wave sleep (Stage 3 and Stage 4) is decreased. Rapid eye movement sleep shows increased α-activity and it was hypothesized that it was due to early disconnection between generators of REM and NREM sleep in PD. It is debated whether REM sleep percentage is normal or reduced. Electromyographic atonia is periodically abolished in REM sleep. Repetitive blinking is seen in the beginning of the recording and blepharospasm is seen during slow wave sleep before the REM sleep episodes. Polysomnography has revolutionized the sleep assessment in PD.

MANAGEMENT

The treatment of insomnia should be preceded by the identification of the type of insomnia and the factors responsible for it. It is necessary to rule out and treat the sleep related breathing and movement disorders if present. It is necessary to alter the therapy if insomnia is due to motor complications L-dopa-carbidopa controlled release preparations[13] ropinirole 24-hour sustained release preparation (2–24 mg/day), transdermal rotigotine patch (up to 16 mg/day) significantly improves nocturnal-akinesia.[14,15] Rasagiline a monoamine oxidase B inhibitor improves insomnia by increasing endogenous melatonin level.[16]

If insomnia is not due to PD motor complications, the principal therapy is cognitive behavioral therapy (CBT), focusing on sleep wake cycle, behavior hygiene, sleep restriction relaxation and cognitive techniques. Various hypnotic drugs like eszopiclone (2–3 mg/day) zolpidem (5–10 mg/day), trazodone (25–75 mg), doxepin (10 mg), ramelteon, and melatonin (3 mg) were tried.[17-20] Nocturia is mainly due to automatic disturbance and the loss of D1-mediated inhibition of micturition associated with detrusor hyperreflexia, subcutaneous apomorphine (3–8 mg), intranasal desmopressin, and botulinum toxin injection into detrusor muscle are not sufficiently proven. Anticholinergic like solifenacin[21] (5–10 mg/day), darifenacin (7.5 mg/day), and tolterodine (2 mg/day) have better tolerability than nonselective drugs like oxybutynin (5 mg/day) and trospium (10–20 mg twice daily).

For RLS, dopamine agonists (DAs) (long acting) pregabalin, gabapentin, low dose opioids can be considered.[22] Dopamine agonists also helps in reducing PLMs.[23]

Clonazepam (0.25–2 mg at hour of sleep) is the first line pharmacological treatment for NREM parasomnia (confusion arousals, sleepwalking, sleep terrors).[24] Rapid eye movement parasomnias (nightmares) is treated by CBT particularly imagery rehearsal therapy (IRT).[25] Rapid eye movement sleep behavioral disorder is better treated by clonazepam (0.25–2 mg) 30 minutes before bedtime. Clonazepam is contraindicated in moderate and severe Obstructive sleep apneas. In such cases melatonin (3–12 mg) before sleep can be tried.[26]

Sleep related breathing disorders are treated by the standard therapy of CPAP(continuous positive airway pressure), weight reduction, sleeping on one side are recently mandibular advancement devices are beneficial in treating obstructive sleep apnea.[27]

Excessive day time sleepiness treatment in PD is a challenge. If patient is treated with L-dopa and DAs, switch DA with rasagiline or selegiline as all DA's cause more EDS than L-dopa. Modafinil (100–400 mg/day) is helpful in Expanded Disability Status Scale. Nocturnally administered sodium oxybate (3–9 mg at hour of sleep) in two split doses (at bedtime and 4 hours later) improve EDS and fatigue in PD. Methylphenidate (1 mg/kg three times daily, for 3 months), caffeine (200 mg/BD) are also tried in treating EDS, but further studies are needed.[28-30]

CONCLUSION

Understanding the sleep problems in PD and their treatment is challenging. An accurate clinical and diagnostic assessment is necessary before initiating treatment. Many treatment options are now available but further randomized controlled trials are needed to confirm their efficacy.

REFERENCES

1. Kumar S, Bhatia M, Behari M. Sleep disorders in Parkinson's disease. Mov Disord. 2002;17(4):775-81.
2. Verbaan D, van Rooden SM, Visser M, et al. Nighttime sleep problems and daytime sleepiness in Parkinson's disease. Mov Disord. 2008;23(1):35-41.
3. Lai EC, Jankovic J, Krauss JK, et al. Long-term efficacy of posteroventral pallidotomy in the treatment of Parkinson's disease. Neurology. 2000;55(8):1218-22.
4. Daroff RB, Jankovic J, Mazziotta JC, Pomeroy SL, Bradley WG (Walter G. Bradley's neurology in clinical practice.
5. Cummings JL. Depression and Parkinson's disease: A review. Am J Psychiatry. 1992;149(4):443-54.
6. Cummings JL. Managing psychosis in patients with Parkinson's disease. N Engl J Med. 1999;340(10):801-3.
7. Shulman LM, Wen X, Weiner WJ, et al. Acupuncture therapy for the symptoms of Parkinson's disease. Mov Disord. 2002;17(4):799-802.
8. Aarsland D, Andersen K, Larsen JP, et al. Prevalence and characteristics of dementia in Parkinson Disease. Arch Neurol. 2003;60(3):387.

9. Chen M-H, Lu C-H, Chen P-C, et al. Association between autonomic impairment and structural deficit in Parkinson disease. Medicine (Baltimore). 2016;95(11):e3086.
10. Lees A, Blackburn N, neuropharmacology VC-C, 1988 undefined. The nighttime problems of Parkinson's disease. europepmc.org [Internet]. [cited 2018 May 30]; Available from: http://europepmc.org/abstract/med/3233589
11. Onofrj M, Luciano A, Thomas A, Neurology DI-, 2003 undefined. Mirtazapine induces REM sleep behavior disorder (RBD) in parkinsonism. AAN Enterp [Internet]. [cited 2018 May 31]; Available from: http://n.neurology.org/content/60/1/113.short
12. Rye DB, Bliwise DL, Dihenia B, et al. Daytime sleepiness in Parkinson's disease. J Sleep Res. 2000;9(1):63-9.
13. Wailke S, Herzog J, Witt K, et al. Effect of controlled-release levodopa on the microstructure of sleep in Parkinson's disease. Eur J Neurol. 2011;18(4):590-6.
14. Ray Chaudhuri K, Martinez-Martin P, Rolfe KA, et al. Improvements in nocturnal symptoms with ropinirole prolonged release in patients with advanced Parkinson's disease. Eur J Neurol. 2012;19(1):105-13.
15. Poewe WH, Rascol O, Quinn N, et al. Efficacy of pramipexole and transdermal rotigotine in advanced Parkinson's disease: A double-blind, double-dummy, randomised controlled trial. Lancet Neurol. 2007;6(6):513-20.
16. Melone MA, Schettino C, Dato C, et al. Rasagiline for sleep disorders in patients with Parkinson's disease: A prospective observational study. Neuropsychiatr Dis Treat. 2016;12:2497-502.
17. Menza M, Dobkin RD, Marin H, et al. Treatment of insomnia in Parkinson's disease: A controlled trial of eszopiclone and placebo. Mov Disord. 2010;25(11):1708-14.
18. Lavoisy J, Marsac J. Zolpidem in Parkinson's disease. Lancet. 1997;350(9070):74.
19. Kashihara K, Nomura T, Maeda T, et al. Beneficial effects of ramelteon on rapid eye movement sleep behavior disorder associated with Parkinson's disease - Results of a multicenter open trial. Intern Med. 2016;55(3):231-6.
20. Medeiros CAM, Carvalhedo de Bruin PF, Lopes LA, et al. Effect of exogenous melatonin on sleep and motor dysfunction in Parkinson's disease. J Neurol. 2007;254(4):459-64.
21. Sakakibara R, Panicker J, Finazzi-Agro E, et al. A guideline for the management of bladder dysfunction in Parkinson's disease and other gait disorders. Neurourol Urodyn. 2016;35(5):551-63.
22. Allen RP, Ondo WG, Ball E, et al. Restless legs syndrome (RLS) augmentation associated with dopamine agonist and levodopa usage in a community sample. Sleep Med. 2011;12(5):431-9.
23. Puligheddu M, Figorilli M, Aricò D, et al. Time structure of leg movement activity during sleep in untreated Parkinson disease and effects of dopaminergic treatment. Sleep Med. 2014;15(7):816-24.
24. Aurora RN, Zak RS, Maganti RK, et al. Best practice guide for the treatment of REM sleep behavior disorder (RBD). J Clin Sleep Med. 2010;6(1):85-95.
25. McCarter SJ, Boswell CL, St. Louis EK, et al. Treatment outcomes in REM sleep behavior disorder. Sleep Med. 2013;14(3):237-42.
26. McGrane IR, Leung JG, St. Louis EK, et al. Melatonin therapy for REM sleep behavior disorder: a critical review of evidence. Sleep Med. 2015;16(1):19-26.
27. Phillips CL, Grunstein RR, Darendeliler MA, et al. Health outcomes of continuous positive airway pressure versus oral appliance treatment for obstructive sleep apnea. Am J Respir Crit Care Med. 2013;187(8):879-87.
28. Ondo WG, Perkins T, Swick T, et al. Sodium oxybate for excessive daytime sleepiness in Parkinson disease. Arch Neurol. 2008;65(10):1337-40.
29. Devos D, Krystkowiak P, Clement F, et al. Improvement of gait by chronic, high doses of methylphenidate in patients with advanced Parkinson's disease. J Neurol Neurosurg Psychiatry. 2007;78(5):470-5.
30. Postuma RB, Lang AE, Munhoz RP, et al. Caffeine for treatment of Parkinson disease: A randomized controlled trial. Neurology. 2012;79(7):651-8.

CHAPTER 8

Approach to Evaluation and Management of Low Back Ache

R Raghavendran

INTRODUCTION

Low back pain is a common cause of disability. The lordotic lumbar spine bears 60–70% of the body weight, resulting in severe symptoms, sometimes even with trivial changes.

Limited healthcare resources unable to meet the ever increasing demands and increasing number of patients with low back ache (LBA) pose a formidable challenge and a daunting task to those involved in managing these patients. Even with vastly advanced imaging and better understanding of spine bio mechanics, there is no consensus on effective management.[1] We fail to identify the cause in 65% of patients. Persisting back pain, poorly correlates with our diagnosis and image findings. Similar imaging abnormalities (Fig. 1) are seen in a patient with severe pain and an asymptomatic individual.[2] Restoring quality of life and ensuring a return to a normal life should be the priority rather than the correction of image findings. An in-depth, logical, and methodical understanding of spine physiology, biomechanics and its pathophysiology is essential for successful management.

EPIDEMIOLOGY

The lifetime prevalence of low back pain is as high as 80%,[3] with more in women than in men, with an annual prevalence rate of around 40%. Prevalence rate increases with age, peaking in the seventh decade. The prevalence is higher in better socioeconomic populations, due to a sedentary lifestyle and obesity. Risk factors associated with an acute pain episode progressing to chronic back pain include psychological stress, compensation conflicts, job dissatisfaction, over and above the pathological nature of the disease. Failure to identify a specific spine disease after an exhaustive historical, clinical and imaging examination, leads to patients being labelled as non-specific LBA. The number of such non-specific LBA patients are on the rise. Hence clinicians need to develop

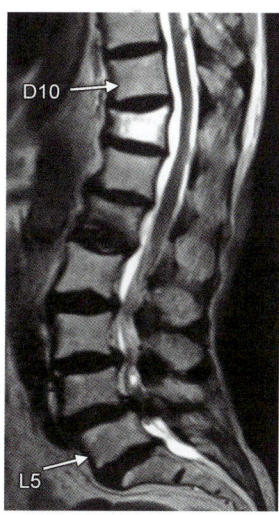

FIG 1: T2 weighted magnetic resonance imaging showing multiple disc herniations, disc migration, exaggeration of lumbar lordosis, old fracture of L1 and spondylolisthesis at L4/L5 with severe lumbar canal stenosis, all in same patient.

an individualized management option for each patient.

APPROACH

Evaluation of LBA needs a thorough understanding about the duration, type, site, precipitating and alleviating factors of the pain, similar previous episodes, family, and medical history and associated systemic signs. A thorough systemic examination is essential. Imaging and lab investigations are primarily guided by the clinical features of the particular individual. The goal is to arrive at a diagnosis which correlates with the signs and symptoms of the patient, with the help of ancillary lab and imaging parameters. Sometimes HPE of the abnormal tissue may be required. The following steps are a guide to establish the diagnosis and proceed with the definitive treatment, medical or surgical.

Evaluation of Pain Etiology

Almost all the anatomical substrates of the spinal column are pain generators resulting in a plethora of varied painful conditions to deal with in LBA (Flowchart 1).[1]

Infective

Pain associated with fever and weight loss may occasionally be associated with radiating pain. Can have delayed neurological deficits. Axial skeletal infective process like vertebral osteomyelitis, discitis, epidural abscess, and granulomas are common conditions. Imaging frequently shows involvement of adjacent disc space and vertebral body. A high degree of suspicion is needed to rule out this condition, because more of than not, it may present with sudden profound neurological deficits that will need emergency surgical procedure.

Neoplastic

Localized spinal pain in recumbent position, often severe, particularly during night time should raise a strong suspicion of neoplastic cause.

Benign lesions: More commonly seen in third decade. Common lesions are osteochondromas, osteoid osteomas, hemangiomas, and aneurysmal bone cysts among others.

Malignant lesions: Metastasis to spine is more common than primary spine malignancy, and is due to direct or hematogenous spread. Autopsy evaluations prove spine as the most common site of skeletal metastasis. Vertebral Body is the most involved part of spine in metastasis. In imaging usually the disc space is preserved and uninvolved. Breast, lung and prostate are the more common primary malignancies that spread to spine. Common primary spine malignancies are multiple myeloma and Ewing's sarcoma. Patients can have rapid neurological deficits and may end up with permanent deficits if diagnosis is delayed.

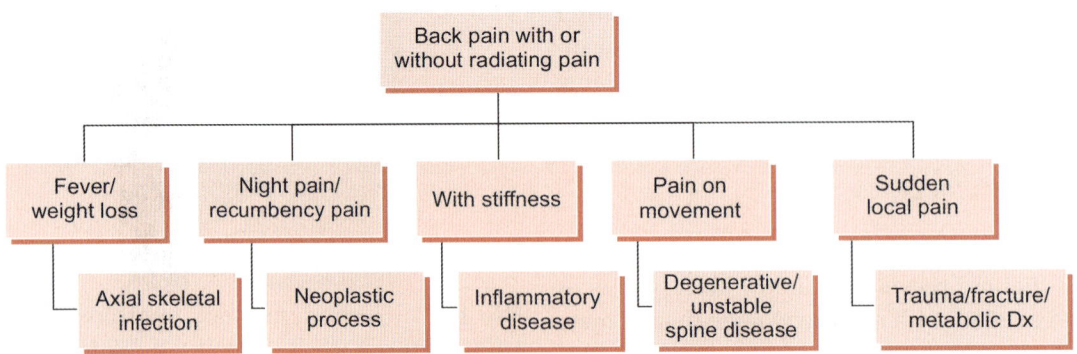

FLOWCHART 1: An algorithm for the approach to a patient with low back pain.

Disc Degeneration

Biochemical aging phenomenon of the disc material is a common image finding in symptomatic as well as asymptomatic patients.[4] Symptoms are often vague. They present with non-specific symptomatology, most commonly nonradiating LBA or with occasional radiation to sacroiliac joints. The image finding does not predict the severity of symptoms. The annulus of degenerated disc undergoes nerve proliferation particularly at the point of annulus breach, and may contribute to severe pain with minimal image changes.

Disc Prolapse (Figs 2 to 5)

Pain is acute in onset classically radiating to the leg (mostly up to the knee and uncommonly up to the foot) on the side of nerve root compression.

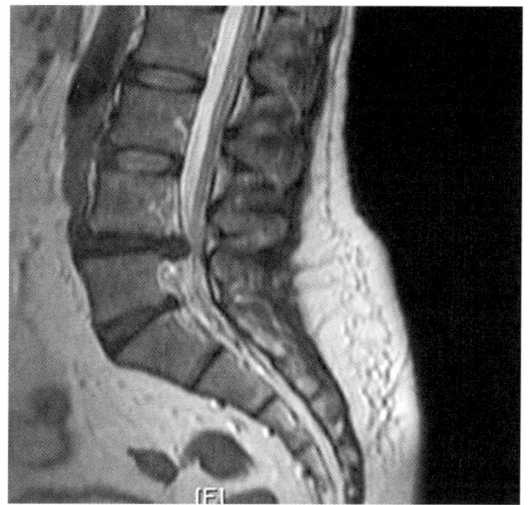

FIG. 2: L4-L5 prolapsed disc material.

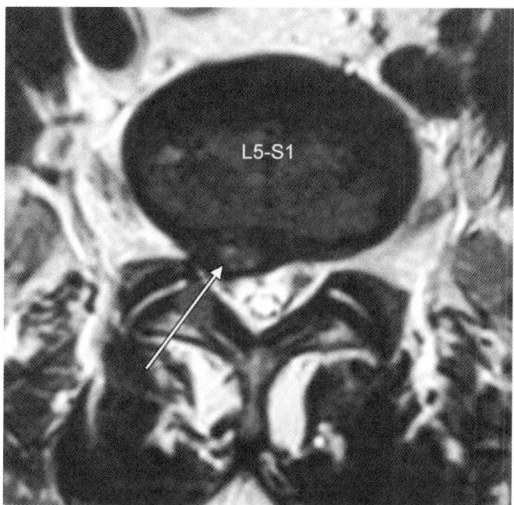

FIG. 4: Magnetic resonance imaging T2 axial view of the L5-S1 intervertebral disc showing a posterolateral disc herniation compressing right S1 nerve root.

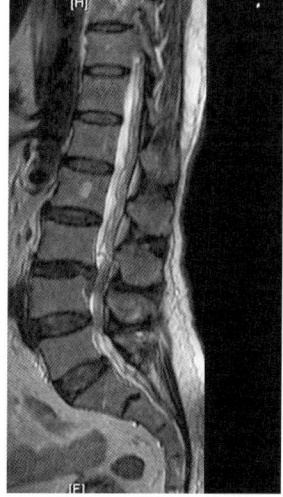

FIG. 3: Magnetic resonance imaging showing an extruded L3-L4 disc with inferior migration (T2 sagittal view).

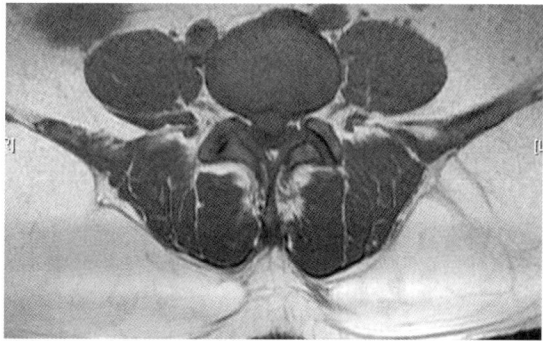

FIG. 5: Magnetic resonance imaging T1 axial view of the L4–L5 intervertebral disc showing a central disc herniation, presented as cauda equina syndrome.

Pain is often reproduced by coughing, sneezing and will increase in severity with activity, weight bearing, flexion, standing, and sitting. Depending on the nerve root affected, patient can have corresponding dermatomal sciatica, paresthesia or myotomal motor weakness.

Posterolateral disc herniation is more common than central disc herniation since the posterior longitudinal ligament is strongest in midline and is weak laterally. Commonly the exiting nerve root beneath the pedicle of inferior vertebra is involved, e.g., L4-L5 disc prolapse will compress L5 nerve root.

Lumbar Canal Stenosis

Gradual onset with slowly progressive symptoms. Patients with single level stenosis present with dermatomal pattern, mimicking a lumbar disc prolapse. Multilevel stenosis present with intermittent neurogenic claudication. A classical claudication presents as pain, numbness or tingling sensation on standing or walking, relieved by sitting, or forward bending. These patients commonly have associated degenerative spondylolisthesis. Lumbar canal stenosis patients have significantly poor quality of life compared to all other causes of LBA.

Spinal Cord Tumors

Extradural and intradural tumors (Figs 6 and 7): Nerve sheath tumors and meningiomas constitute 75% of this category. Adults most commonly present with diffuse, nocturnal back pain not relieved with rest,[5] whereas in children the presentation is gait and motor disturbances. Long-standing patients will have lower limb weakness with or without bladder-bowel involvement.

Inflammatory

Severe persistent axial stiffness and pain reducing with increased mechanical activity is a classical presentation of inflammatory pathology. Rheumatoid arthritis and ankylosing Spondylitis are the most common inflammatory illness. Neurological deficits are very rare.

Degenerative Spine Problems—Instability Pain

Classically pain without constitutional symptoms and exacerbates with activity.

Spondylolysis (Fig. 8) and consequent spondylolisthesis (Figs 9 and 10) are the most common conditions.[6] Other causes include facet joint arthropathy and congenital

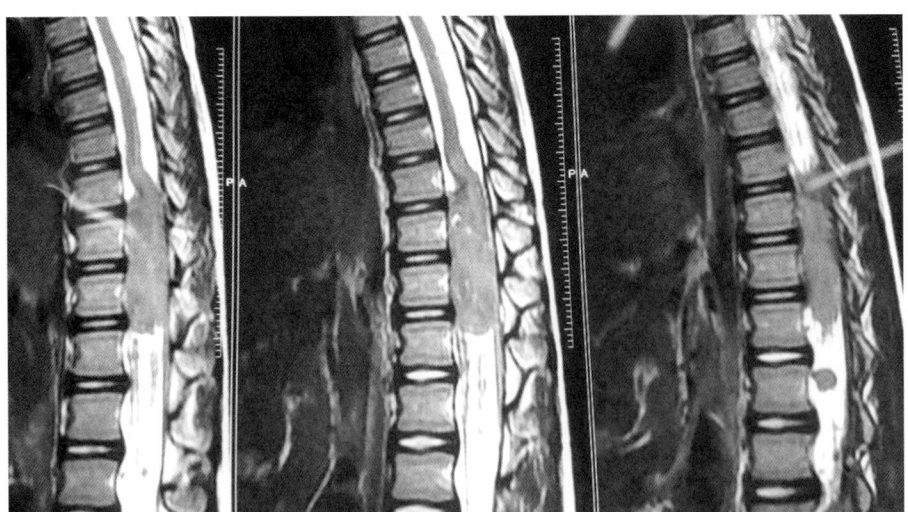

FIG. 6: Sagittal T2 weighted magnetic resonance imaging showing an intramedullary tumor, excision revealed an astrocytoma.

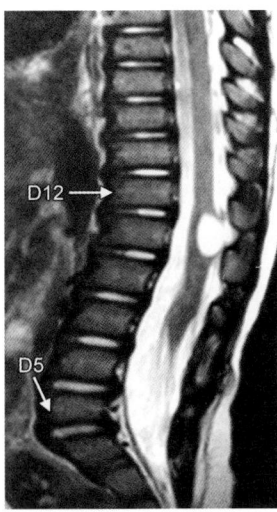

FIG. 7: Sagittal T2 weighted magnetic resonance imaging showing a benign arachnoid cyst at L1 level.

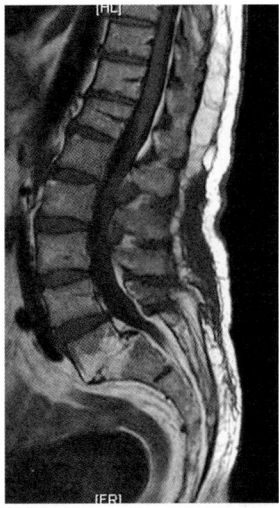

FIG. 9: T1 weighted magnetic resonance imaging of a patient with grade 2 anterolisthesis. Also note the signal intensity changes in the end plates and marrow of L5 and S1.

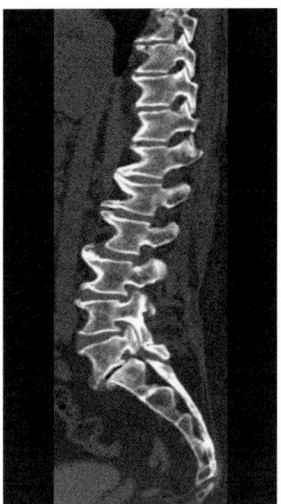

FIG. 8: Sagittal computed tomography showing a grade 1 spondylolisthesis of L5 over S1 with extensive spondylotic, degenerative changes and osteophyte formation with vacuum phenomenon (air in the disc space) at L5/S1.

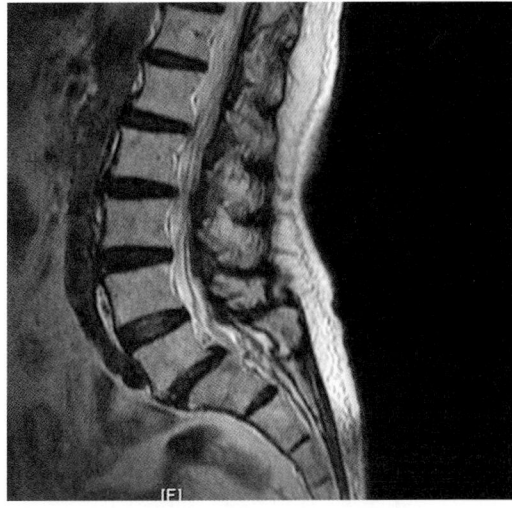

FIG. 10: Grade 1 L5–S1 anterolisthesis with apparent disc herniation and superior migration of disc material.

conditions like sacralization or lumbarization and congenital pars interarticularis defect. Pain is relieved completely with rest. History of trauma is often present. Spondylolysis is defect in pars interarticularis either unilateral or bilateral. Most commonly spondylolysis is seen in L5 level, resulting in L5-S1 level, being the commonest spondylolisthesis.

Trauma

Localized acute pain associated with tenderness is always considered due to trauma. Pain

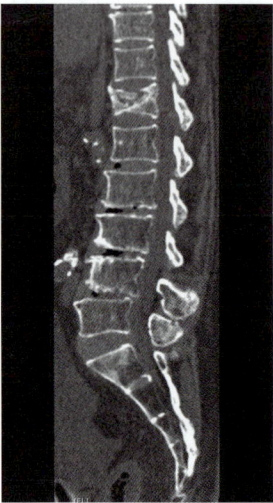

FIG. 11: Sagittal computed tomography image showing a D12 wedge compression fracture with vacuum phenomenon at multiple disc levels with degenerative L4-L5 retrolisthesis.

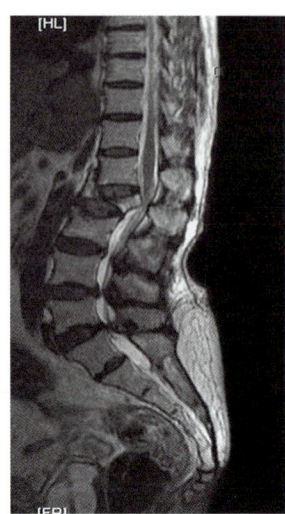

FIG. 13: Sagittal T2-weighted magnetic resonance imaging showing L1 fracture with retropulsion of fragments and severe canal compromise.

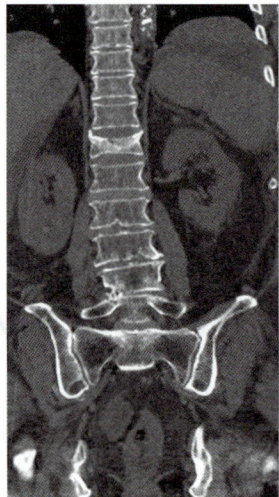

FIG. 12: Coronal computed tomography image showing D12 fracture.

due to spine trauma is often associated with neurological deficit corresponding to the segmental tenderness with external signs of injury. Fracture (Figs 11 to 13) or ligamentous injury should be suspected until proven otherwise.

Metabolic Disorders

Common metabolic problems like osteoporosis, osteomalacia and Paget's disease affect bone mineralization or density and manifest as localized pain, pathologic vertebral column fractures, or as symptomatic neural entrapments. Systemic signs and symptoms of the disorder are usually detected before the discovery of spine problem.

CLINICAL EXAMINATION

Defining the location, characteristics, and distribution of pain and localization of the neurological deficit requires knowledge about low back pain presentations in combination with lab, electrophysiology, and radiographic imaging results.

Tenderness and Muscle Spasm

Observation of gait, posture, lower back and percussion of the spinous process, greater trochanters, and paraspinal region is done to assess region of maximum tenderness and muscle spasm. Spasm of thigh and leg muscles should also be assessed. Evaluating the region of muscle spasm will give inputs about severity and location of the pathological process.[7] The available range of movement of the spine should be assessed along with normal degree of movement for that age should be defined particularly in anteroposterior plane. Presence of a stepladder deformity or abnormal prominence of the spinous process indicates spondylolisthesis. Tenderness may be absent in chronic spondylolisthesis.

Sacroiliac Joint Tenderness

Tenderness in the anatomically dipped paraspinal region above the gluteal region associated with scoliosis indicates sacroiliac joint pathology.

Hip Joint

Severe pain is elicited while performing the FABER (flexion, abduction, and external rotation) test or a pelvic compression test in case of unilateral or bilateral hip joint pathology.

Posture and Alignment Changes

Body and pelvis tilts away from the pain site and the ipsilateral hip is prominent and elevated in severe painful state. Patients prefer to walk in small steps attempting to keep the knee stiff.

Straight Leg Raising (Lasegue's Sign) Test

Reproduction of sciatic pain between 30 and 70 degrees on passively elevating a hip flexed and knee extended leg, is considered positive for ipsilateral nerve root compression due to a lumbar disc herniation, with a high sensitivity of above 90%, but with low specificity.

Similar sciatic pain in the ipsilateral lower limb on elevating the contralateral leg is known as crossed straight leg raise (Fajersztajn's crossed sciatic sign) which has a high specificity of 88%, though not very sensitive.

Increase in severity and intensity of pain on dorsiflexion of foot (Bragard's sign) or of the big toe (Sicard's sign) while performing Lasegue's test is suggestive of stretch of tibial portion of sciatic nerve.

NEUROLOGICAL EXAMINATION

A complete and thorough neurological examination is very helpful to evaluate the deficit present, progression of the deficit and most importantly to prognosticate the final outcome of the disease. Chronological assessment of the deficit (Flowchart 2) combined with pain characteristics and local examination will invariably clinch the diagnosis even before radiographic imaging is seen, if performed properly. It is rare for a patient with LBA to present with upper motor neuron or myelopathy features, but should be ruled out by a diligent examination. It is very important that the clinical signs and symptoms correlate with the radiological image findings.

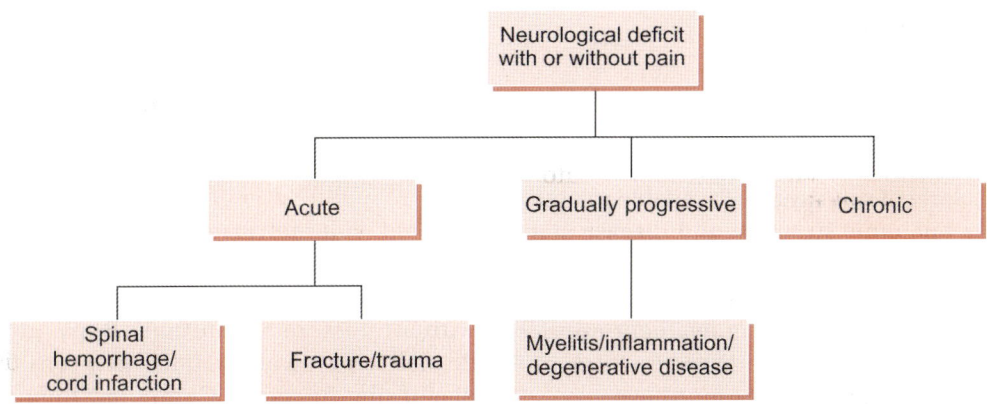

FLOWCHART 2: Flowchart depicting possible etiological approach to a patient with a neurological deficit, with or without back pain.

Each and every nerve root (both sides) is examined separately for its autonomic sensory zone and the myotomal weakness pattern and documented. Subtle bladder and bowel disturbance history is elicited. Acute back pain due to sudden significant disc herniation can present as cauda equina syndrome in which case an urgent surgical decompression should be performed. The examination must include evaluation of brain, brainstem, and spinal cord functions.

PSYCHOLOGICAL SCREENING

Chronic low back pain patients often suffer from depression. Depression and stress are proved factors that exacerbate pain and affect the final outcome adversely.

Psychological assessment should be an integral part of evaluating LBA patients, particularly those in whom surgery is contemplated.

IMAGING OF SPINE

Radiographic imaging is critical to the management of LBA. Magnetic resonance imaging (MRI), computed tomography (CT), and plain radiographs are used in conjunction with clinical data to confirm or refute the presumed diagnosis. Imaging changes are common in asymptomatic patients also. The strength and weakness of each imaging modality should be understood and interpreted accordingly to decide on an appropriate treatment protocol.

Magnetic Resonance Imaging

It is the initial imaging technique performed on all LBA patients whatever the clinical diagnosis. Highly detailed visualization of spine anatomy (particularly of soft tissue) is available to assess specific anatomic structure and disease state. In traumatic situations MRI gives information to classify as well as manage patients with spinal cord injury, extent of ligament injuries, differentiate chronic from acute fracture, and identify disc herniation or hemorrhage.

T1 imaging: Demonstrates vertebral bodies, intervertebral disc, nerve roots, tumors, and spinal cord clearly. Contrast T1 is useful to diagnose infectious, inflammatory lesions and tumors.

T2 imaging: It clearly differentiates normal from abnormal anatomy. Cerebrospinal fluid (CSF), cysts, intervertebral disc, infections, and tumors are easily distinguished.

Diffusion-weighted Imaging

Has a limited role in evaluation of spine pathology. Absent diffusion restriction in degenerative disc is helpful to differentiate it from infectious pathology. Decreased apparent diffusion coefficient values seen in dorsal root ganglion of the affected nerve root following disc herniation predicts poor recovery of symptoms in patients.

Diffusion Tensor Imaging

Diffusion tensor imaging (DTI) detects signal changes even when T1 and T2 are normal. In myelopathy patients DTI indices differentiate symptomatic from asymptomatic individuals with cord compression. The DTI tractography detects spinal cord fiber involvement and determines surgical planning and resectability of tumors.

Susceptibility-weighted Imaging

Depicts spine arteriovenous anatomy without the need for contrast. Highly sensitive in detecting small hemorrhages both traumatic and spontaneous.

Magnetic resonance imaging chemical shift imaging Dixon and magnetic resonance neurography are valuable recent additions to the MRI evaluation of LBA.

Computed Tomography

A rapid volumetric acquisition is possible with multi detector CT, enabling concurrent evaluation of spine as well as other body regions without loss of resolution. Bony anatomy delineation is excellent. It has 98% sensitivity in diagnosing fractures. Computed tomography accurately defines bone quality, size of implants and adequacy of spinal elements in

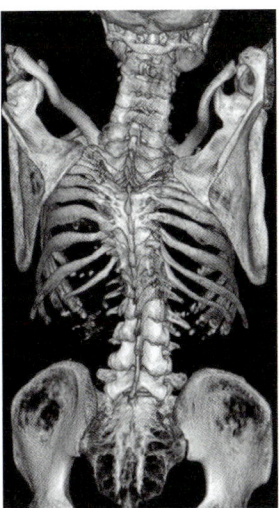

FIG 14: 3D reconstructed computed tomography image exquisitely demonstrating kyphoscoliosis.
(For color version, see Plate 5)

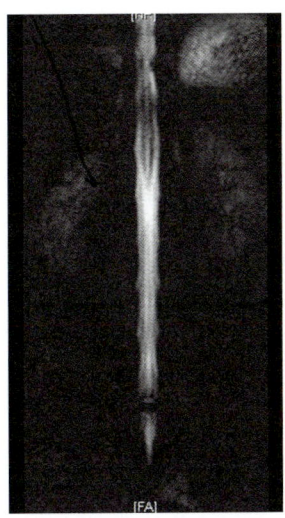

FIG 15: Coronal magnetic resonance myelogram showing complete cerebrospinal fluid block at L5-S1 level.

patients planned for spine instrumentation. In hemodynamically unstable trauma patients the ability of CT to acquire images rapidly with a high negative predictive value is a choice to rule out spine injury compared to time consuming MRI. Positron emission tomography CT is useful in evaluating neoplastic and infectious spinal diseases.

Plain Radiographs

Rapidly obtained, widely available and relatively inexpensive, plain radiographs have a very important role in assessment of low back pain. It is most valuable to evaluate the bony alignment, graft and instrumentation position, abnormal motion of vertebrae in flexion and extension, to assess stability in traumatic and pathological fractures and ligament disruptions, and also spondylolisthesis during weight bearing. Postoperative radiographs are useful to evaluate instrumentation position.

Myelography

Performed by injecting contrast agent into thecal space. Magnetic resonance myelography (Figs 15 and 16) obtained non- invasively is also useful. Typical indications for CT myelography are for patients with implants

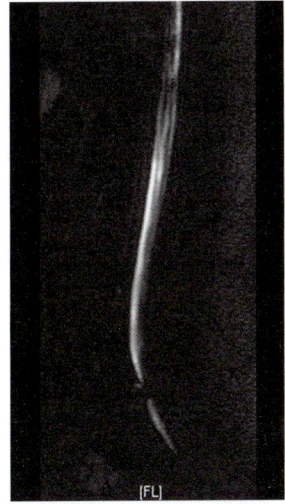

FIG 16: Sagittal magnetic resonance myelogram of the same patient showing complete cerebrospinal fluid block.

not MRI compatible (e.g., pacemaker), unclear image due to presence of metallic implants, those suffering from claustrophobia and patients with high degree of kyphoscoliosis which makes acquisition and interpretation of images difficult. Computed tomography myelography (5–7%) more accurately evaluates lateral recess anatomy in cases of nerve root compression in lumbar disc herniation and lumbar canal stenosis, compared to MRI which can overestimate nerve root compression and canal stenosis by almost 30%.

Computed tomography myelography is the most sensitive tool in establishing the presence of CSF leak. It is a helpful adjunct in planning targeted epidural blood patch, fibrin glue treatment or possible surgical repair of CSF leaks. The sensitivity of CT myelography to detect nerve root avulsion is 100%, whereas MRI has 88% sensitivity.

Nuclear Scans

A useful screening tool for known patients of malignancy. In spinal infections used in conjunction with other cross-section imaging modalities to differentiate infectious from degenerative pathology. Nuclear scans are useful in detecting implant loosening and pseudoarthrosis.

Ultrasonography

Has limited use in spine problems. Mainly useful in pediatric spinal dysraphism. Useful tool intra-operatively to delineate lesion-cord interface, differentiate solid from cystic components in tumours and intraoperatively reveal lesions difficult to visualize during surgery.

CORRELATION OF IMAGE AND CLINICAL FINDINGS

After obtaining appropriate imaging, the findings must be interpreted in clinical context. Correlating image findings with clinical picture is challenging because, frequently radiographic interpretations contain pathological findings like disc bulge or protrusion, Schmorl's nodes, annular tears, end plate changes, facet arthropathy, foraminal stenosis and disc degeneration in both symptomatic as well as asymptomatic patients. In patients without deformity or neural element compression, surgical intervention based on MRI degenerative changes has proved to be not beneficial. Patients with worsening neurological deficits should undergo MRI irrespective of findings in other imaging modalities. Before a decision about management of LBA is made, it is important that correlation of image finding with clinical picture is absolute and be sure that the radiographic findings are indeed the true cause of LBA.

ELECTROPHYSIOLOGICAL STUDIES

Sensory-evoked potentials and motor-evoked potentials have been shown to be useful in predicting adverse neurological outcomes in patients with LBA. Intraoperative neuro monitoring is an established effective tool to alert the surgeon, as well as predict an increased risk of paraperesis and paraplegia in the postoperative period. It is an integral part of many surgeon's practice.

MANAGEMENT OF LOW BACK ACHE

The initial management of LBA is a right combination of pharmacotherapy, graded and monitored physical activity, cognitive behavior modifications, and rehabilitation.[11] The utility of interventional procedures like epidural and facet joint steroid injections is unclear and controversial. Available evidence suggests that prolonged bed rest and polypharmacy involving narcotics and muscle relaxants should be avoided.

Pharmacological Management

Initially a short course of analgesia mainly NSAIDs (acetaminophen) and exercise along with life style modifications is started.[8] Judicious usage of weak opioids and muscle relaxants maybe beneficial but should be used with caution. Antidepressants are helpful in managing coincident depression. Pharmacological therapy should be often re-evaluated and changed according to the symptom changes noted.[9]

Nonpharmacological Treatment

Chronic LBA patients benefit with therapeutic massage, ultrasonography, exercise therapy and spinal manipulation. In acute painful episode evidence supports only the use of superficial heat as beneficial compared to laser, lumbar support, short wave diathermy, transcutaneous nerve stimulation and ultrasonography. In LBA patients with or without sciatica, prolonged bed rest is known to increase pain and reduce function when compared to unrestricted activities.

Behavioral therapy is beneficial than usual care in patients with high-risk psychological factors for developing chronic LBA. Yoga and exercise therapies are beneficial in treatment of LBA. The benefit is more if they are combined with concurrent educational sessions of these modalities.[10]

Spinal manipulations, acupuncture, and physical interventions found limited or no evidence to show they are beneficial compared to usual care. Reduced self-reporting of pain and improved functions are noted, but not a meaningful difference when compared to usual care alone.

Radiation Therapy

Radiation has been very useful adjunct in alleviating low back pain due to metastatic and some primary malignant lesions.

Interventional Therapy

Evidence recommends against the use of facet joint steroid injections in nonradiating low back pain. Evidence to suggest recommendations about interlaminar epidural steroid and sacroiliac joint injections is not available. Transforaminal epidural steroid injections may offer benefit in patients with radiculopathy due to lumbar disc herniation. The available evidence do not support interventional therapies in the treatment of long standing LBA.

Surgery

The clear indications for surgery are:
- Failed appropriate conservative therapy with a surgically treatable cause
- Incapacitating pain interfering with daily activities due to a surgically correctable pathology as in lumbar disc herniations
- Persistent or worsening neurological deficit or identifying a fresh deficit in a chronic patient
- To prevent impending neurological deficit when clinical and imaging evidence indicate progression of the disease as in tumors, infective, unstable spine, etc.
- To obtain histopathological diagnosis as in infective or neoplastic lesions
- Correction and restoration of spinal alignment with instrumentation in cases of spondylolysis, spondylolisthesis, etc.
- To correct instability of spine and consequent pain reduction as in case of fracture stabilization and also in spondylolisthesis.

Surgery being a definitive treatment in management of LBA, patient selection, correlation of radiologic and clinical findings, establishing that the image finding needing surgically corrective measures is undoubtedly the cause of LBA and that the surgical procedure planned will give complete relief of symptoms to the patient. The goal should be alleviating pain of the patient rather than correction of image findings. Carefully selected patients who underwent the appropriate surgical procedure have had a satisfying and comfortable pain free lifestyle compared with those operated on improper selection criteria.

CONCLUSION

Carefully graded evidence based guidelines combining the use of effective and safe pharmacological interventional therapies, patient specific selection of candidates for surgical intervention and appropriately designed surgical procedure results in achieving optimal outcomes. The main goal of approaching these patients is to restore the functional outcome of the patient with minimum of interventions.

REFERENCES

1. Biyani A, Andersson GBJ. Low back pain: Pathophysiology and management. J Am Acad Orthop Surg. 2004;12(2):106-15.
2. van Tulder MW, Assendelft WJ, Koes BW, et al. Spinal radiographic findings and nonspecific low back pain.

A systematic review of observational studies. Spine (Phila Pa 1976). 1997;22(4):427-34.
3. Cherkin DC, Deyo RA, Wheeler K, et al. Physician views about treating low back pain. The results of a national survey. Spine (Phila Pa 1976). 1995;20(1):1-9; discussion 9-10.
4. Seitsalo S, Schlenzka D, Poussa M, et al. Disc degeneration in young patients with isthmic spondylolisthesis treated operatively or conservatively: A long-term follow-up. Eur Spine J. 1997; 6(6): 393-7.
5. Tobias ME, McGirt MJ, Chaichana KL, et al. Surgical management of long intramedullary spinal cord tumors. Child's Nerv Syst. 2008;24(2):219-23.
6. Saraste H. Spondylolysis and spondylolisthesis. Acta Orthopaedica Scandinavica. 1993;64: 84-6.
7. Lesher JM, Dreyfuss P, Hager N, et al. Hip joint pain referral patterns: A descriptive study. Pain Med. 2008;9(1):22-5.
8. Malmivaara A, Häkkinen U, Aro T, et al. The treatment of acute low back pain--bed rest, exercise therapy or ordinary activity? N Engl J Med. 1995;332(6):351-5.
9. American Society of Anesthesiologists Task Force on Chronic Pain Management; American Society of Regional Anesthesia and Pain Medicine. Practice guidelines for chronic pain management: An updated report by the American Society of Anesthesiologists task force on chronic pain management and the American Society of Regional Anesthesia and Pain Medicine. Anesthesiology. 2010;112(4):810-33.
10. Kamper SJ, Apeldoorn AT, Chiarotto A, et al. Multidisciplinary biopsychosocial rehabilitation for chronic low back pain. Cochrane Database Syst Rev. 2014;(9):CD000963.
11. Guzmán J, Esmail R, Karjalainen K, et al. Multidisciplinary rehabilitation for chronic low back pain: Systematic review. BMJ. 2001;322(7301):1511-6.

CHAPTER 9

Management of Parkinson Disease in This Millennium

Goutam KA, AV Srinivasan, Poorna J Visa, V Rajalakshmi

INTRODUCTION

By the year 2040, neurodegenerative disease are expected to surpass cancer as the second most common cause of death in the elderly. One of the most neurodegenerative disorder in Parkinsons' disease (PD), with over 4 million victims identified world-wide. Aging has been implicated as an important risk for PD, with the majority of cases occurring in people above the age of 60 years. Now that our population is experiencing an extended lifespan, the prevalence of Parkinson's disease is likely to increase substantially. Indeed, it is estimated that one in 40 persons will develop this disease.

Parkinson's disease was described by James Parkinson in 1817 as a clinical syndrome presenting with bradykinesia, tremor and slow, shuffling gait with postural instability. Rigidity was described later, but is included as a key clinical feature in the current diagnosis makes up approximately 80% of case of Parkinsonism.[1]

Definition

Characteristic tetrad known as TRAP
- Resting tremor
- Cogwheel rigidity
- Bradykinesia/akinesia
- Postural reflexes.

Of this tetrad, only resting tremor is truly suggestive of PD, an early sign that may remain prominent even late in the disorder.[2] The others occur in varying degrees in other forms of Parkinsonism.

Diagnostic Criteria

The gold standard for diagnosis of PD remains then neuropathological examination. There is still no biological marker that unequivocally confirms the diagnosis.

In autopsy studies a final diagnosis of PD before death has been incorrect in about 24% of cases.

Clinical diagnostic criteria: Bradykinesia (slowness of initiation of voluntary movement with progressive reduction in speed and amplitude of respective action) and at least one of the following:
- Muscular rigidity
- 4–6 Hz rest tremor
- Postural instability not caused by primary visual, vestibular, cerebellar, or proprioceptive dysfunction.

Exclusive criteria for Parkinson's disease:
- History of repeated strokes: Stepwise progression of Parkinsonian features
- History of repeated head injury
- History of definite encephalitis
- Oculogyric crisis
- Neuroleptic treatment at onset of symptoms
- Sustained remission
- Strictly unilateral features after 3 years
- Supranuclear gaze palsy
- Cerebellar signs
- Early severe autonomic involvement
- Early severe dementia with disturbance of memory, language and praxis
- Babinski sign

- Presence of cerebral tumor of communicating hydrocephalus on CT scan
- Negative response to large doses of levodopa (L-dopa) (if malabsorption excluded)
- MPTP (1-methyl-4-phenyl-1,2,3,6-tetrahydropyridine) exposure.

Supportive prospective positive criteria for Parkinson's disease: Three or more required for diagnosis of definite PD.
- Unilateral onset
- Rest tremor present
- Progressive disorder
- Persistent asymmetry, affecting side of onset most
- Excellent response to L-dopa
- Severe L-dopa induced chorea
- Levodopa response for 5 years or more
- Clinical course of 10 years or more.

NATIONAL INSTITUTE OF NEUROLOGICAL DISORDERS AND STROKE DIAGONISTIC CRITERIA FOR PARKINSON'S DISEASE

Group A: Features characteristic of PD.
- Resting tremor
- Bradykinesia
- Rigidity
- Asymmetric onset.

Group B: Features suggesting alternative diagnoses.
- Features not usually seen early in the clinical course of PD
- Prominent postural instability in the first 3 years after symptom onset supranuclear gaze palsy (other than restricted upward gaze) or slowing of vertical saccades
   - Freezing phenomenon in the first 3 years
   - Hallucinations unrelated to the medications in the first year
   - Dementia preceding motor symptoms Or in the 1st year
- Severe, symptomatic dysautonomia unrelated to medications
- Documentation of a condition known to produce Parkinsonism

Criteria for possible PD:
- At least two of four features in group A; at least one of these is tremor or bradykinesia
- Either none of the features in group B or symptoms have been present <3 years and none of the features in group B
- Either substantial and sustained response to L-dopa or a dopamine (DA) agonist. Patient has not had adequate trial of L-dopa or a DA agonist.

Criteria for possible PD: At least three of the four features in group A are present and none of the features in group B (symptom duration of at least 3 years is necessary) and substantial and sustained response to L-dopa or a DA agonist.

Criteria for definite PD: All criteria for possible PD are met and histopathologic confirmation.

EPIDEMIOLOGY

As a rule Parkinsons' disease (PD) begins between the ages of 40 and 70, with peak age at onset occurring in the sixth decade. Onset at younger than age 20 is known as juvenile Parkinsonism, which has a different pattern of nigral degeneration and is often hereditary (parkin-gene) or caused by Huntington's or Wilson's disease. PD is more common in men, with a male-to-female ratio of 3:2.[3]

Parkinson's disease makes up approximately 80% of cases of Parkinsonism. The prevalence of PD is approximately 160 cases per 100,000 population, and the incidence is about 20 cases per 100,000 population.[3] However, both prevalence and incidence with age; at age 70 years, reach approximately 55–120 cases per 100,000 population per year respectively.[3]

The incidence in all countries where vital statistics are kept is the same. Considering this frequency, coincidence in a family on the basis of chance occurrence might be as high as 5%

Etiological Factors

The exact cause of PD remains unclear. A combination of factors probably is responsible for development of PD. Various theories include the following.[4]

Accelerated Aging

- Normal aging is associated with clinical features that may resemble PD

- Aging is associated with a decline of pigmented neurons in the substantia nigra and with decreased levels of striatal DA and dopa decarboxylase
- Some authorities believe that PD may result from the effects of aging superimposed on an insult to the nigrostriatal system earlier in life.

Oxidative Stress
- This theory receives much support and attention in recent literature. PD patients may suffer the combined effects of multiple factors culminating in damage from free radicals
- Parkinsons' disease patients may suffer the combined effects of multiple factors culminating in damage from free radicals
- Dopamine oxidation can result in formation of hydrogen peroxide, as well as the superoxide anion radical
- Hydrogen peroxide can undergo reactions with ferrous ions, resulting in formation of the highly toxic hydroxyl radical
- These hydroxyl radicals can cause cell membrane damage.

Genetic Susceptibility
- Twin studies have often proven inconclusive
- Genetic factors seem to play a greater role in PD with earlier onset
- An increased incidence of a family history of PD is observed in affected individuals (16% vs. 4% controls).

Environmental Toxins
- Cyanide
- Manganese
- Carbon disulfide
- Pesticides
- Well water
- Methanol
- Organic solvents

Medications
- Metoclopramide
- Domperidone
- Reserpine containing antihypertensives
- Neuroleptics

Natural History

The pathological changes of PD may appear as much as three decades before the appearance of clinical signs. Onset is so gradual and insidious, however, that patients rarely can pinpoint the first symptom(s). Early symptoms may be so mild that a clinical diagnosis is not possible.

A large body of evidence indicates the progression of PD may be rapid in the preclinical stage as well as during the first years of the disease, with subsequent slowing of progress.[5.]

In this profile of clinical, biochemical and pathological changes in PD, the brain's compensating mechanisms are seen to be increase in the synthesis of DA receptors and turnovers of surviving the necrosis (SN) reflected by an increase in the homovanillic acid (HVA), DA ratio.

Before the introduction of L-DOPA, PD cause severe disability in 16% of patients with 5 years of onset in 37% of during the next 5 years, and in 42% of those surviving of 15 years.

The motor cause of PD is characterized by a preclinical phase during which neuronal degeneration progresses, but compensatory mechanisms allow normal function. Once clinical symptoms appear, the diagnosis is reached after some variable interval. The early phase of the illness is marked by progressive but mild disability followed by improvement and a stable response to symptomatic therapy.

Advanced PD is characterized by the gradual replacement of the smooth terrain of L-dopa response by an increasingly complex landscape of motor fluctuations. A panoply of nonmotor symptoms and signs add to the management complexity.

During the early years of L-dopa treatment, patients should be questioned routinely about signs of "wearing off" response or dyskinesia. Specifically each patient should be asked about return of minimal tremor, bradykinesia, voice softness, or decreased manual dexterity after a dose of L-dopa[6]

Motor abnormalities are influenced by peripheral and central L-dopa pharmacokinetics and central pharmacodynamaic influences.

Consulations: Most commonly requested consultations are with neurologists, neuosurgeons, and psychiatrists.
- Consult with a neurologist for
  - Initiation and management of medical therapy
  - Access to clinical medication trials if patients desires, and
  - Management of side effects of L-dopa therapy.
- Consultation with a neurosurgeon may be indicated for a surgical opinion in patients who are resistant to standard medical therapy or who develop significant complications secondary to L-dopa therapy.
- Consult a psychiatrist for management of depression in patients who do not respond to typical treatment opinions, such as selective serotonin reuptake inhibitors (SSRIs), or who show evidence of contemplating suicide.

Advanced Parkinson's Disease—Pharmacological Management

Motor Problems

Motor Fluctuations

The presence of motor fluctuations decreases the quality of life of PD patients and contributes to the direct and indirect economic burden of the disease, reducing occupational productivity and increasing the cost of medical care.

Possible mechanism of L-dopa related motor fluctuations.[7]
- Peripheral Pharmacokinetics:
  - Delayed gastric emptying
  - Protein competition
- Central pharmacokinetics:
  - Variations in striatal L-dopa levels (reduced storage)
  - Damage to dopaminergic neuron by toxic byproducts of DA metabolism
- Central pharmacodynamics:
  - Alleged DA receptors
  - Altered DA receptor sensitivity profile.

Freezing

Considered to be a type of akinesia, freezing takes many forms. Patients may have difficulty with starting to walk (start hesitation) they may suddenly 'freeze' in doorways, while crossing the street, and on turning. The problem may occur at any time, is worsened by stress, any may result in falls.

Freezing may occur during either "on" or "off" states. "On' freezing is poorly understood, and although 'off' freezing is a manifestation of PD, unlike the other characteristics signs, it does not respond readily to L-dopa.

Gait Disturbance

Postural inability is one of the cardinal features of relatively advanced PD. This symptom does not respond to L-dopa.

A focused approach to gait disorders involves. Hesitation when starting to walk (start hesitation) and the temporary inability to move (freezing) can sometimes be overcome by issuing verbal commands ("ready, set, go")

Patients with postural inability may being walking with a few involuntary steps backward. Since these patients have a tendency to fall, their shoes should have leather, not rubber, soles and heel lifts to help tilt then forward.

Other Motor Abnormalities

- Severe burning pain (like fresh sunburn), which as misdiagnoses as fibrositis and was relieved by carbidopa/L-dopa.
- Restless legs, accompanied by kicking and shaking which occurred at regular intervals at the end of each carbidopa/L-dopa dose; symptoms resolved with a change to the CR form.

Nonmotor Problems

Dementia

The dementia associated with PD has been estimated at least 20% of patients, with prevalence higher in order patients and rare in those with younger-onset disease.

Dementia is associated with a poorer prognosis for survival in Parkinson's patients. These patients respond to poorly to L-dopa and experience frequent side effects.

Before treating PD related dementia, it is crucial to eliminate all reversible causes of dementia, such as

- Vitamin B12 deficiency
- Hypothyroidism
- Neurosyphilis
- Normal-pressure hydrocephalus
- Mass lesions.

Depression

An estimated 40–60% of PD patients experience depression, which appears to be related to duration of disease. Whether depression is related to the loss of frontal dopaminergic projections or serotonin deficiency or is a psychological response to PD has not yet been resolved. However, depression is clearly related to the "off" periods of L-dopa response and lifts with improved control of motor symptoms.

Treatment:
- Antidepressant use
- Stimulating antidepressant if apathy is major feature
- Sedating antidepressants if sleep disturbance is major feature

Apathy

In a survey from Norway psychiatric features of PD, it was found that apathy was a significant features affecting these patients.

Although apathy is often confused with depression, it is likely a separate symptom. The most important aspect is to realize that the patient is not "lazy" but that there is a neurologic basis underlying this phenomenon.
- Increase activity
- Caffeine
- Modafinil.

Hallucinations and Psychosis

Psychiatric adverse effects are much more likely to occur in patients with predisposing characteristics such as:
- Dementia
- Advanced age
- Premorbid psychiatric illness
- Exposure to high daily doses of L-dopa.[8]

Visual hallucinations are the most common clinical feature of drug-induced psychosis and occur in approximately 30% of treated patients.

Possible precipitating events include:
- Urinary and pulmonary infections
- Metabolic encephalopathy
- Cerebrovascular events.

Treatment:
- Reduce or stop (medications responsible for symptoms)
- Adjunctive medications (e.g., amantadine, anticholinergics)
- Dopamine agonist
- Catechol-O-methyltransferase inhibitor
- Reduce dosage or L-dopa
- Clozapine
- Quetiapine.

Sleep Disorders

The earliest sleep problem is sleep fragmentation. Sleep problems include difficulty initiating sleep, daytime somnolence, restless legs syndrome (RLS), rapid eye movement (REM) behavior disorders (RBD) sleep apnea (atypical parkinsonism) nightmares, hallucination, dyskinesias, nocturnal Parkinsonism, or dementia-altered sleep-wake cycle.

Sleep Fragmentation

- Controlled-release carbidopa/L-dopa
- Sedating antidepressant
- Clonazepam.

Nocturnal vocalization/vivid dreams: rapid eye movement behavior disorders
- Reduce dopaminergic medications near bedtime
- Clonazepam.

Orthostatic Hypertension

Many patients with PD suffer from orthostatic hypertension, caused either by the disease itself or by the medications used to treat it.

A number of pharmacologic agents are directed at increasing blood pressure (BP). They include the mineralocorticoids. The mineralocorticoids are likely to take several weeks to become effective. A suggested dosing schedule of fludrocortisone (florinef) is 0.2 mg/day, increased to 0.4 mg/day.

Another appropriate option is α1- adrenergic receptor agonist midodrine (ProAmatine). Dosage and administration of midodrine are:
- *Starting dose*: 2.5 mg at breakfast and lunch
- Increase by 2.5 mg increments daily, with minimum 10 mg tid
- Can be given at 3 hour intervals if needed by not more frequently.

Gastrointestinal Problems

Nausea is a recognized, relatively common side effect of all dopaminergic agents. Taking carbidopa, L-dopa with food is sometimes helpful. Should nausea remain a problem, a peripheral DA blocking agent such as domperidone, which does not cross the blood brain barrier, has been found to be extremely effective in reducing both nausea and postural hypotension.

Constipation autonomic dysfunction causing impaired gut motility is common place in PD. Constipation continues to be one of the most frequent autonomic related complaints throughout the disease process.
- High fiber diet, hydration, and exercise program and regularly scheduled toileting are encouraged
- Anticholinergics and narcotic containing compounds should be avoided
- Bulk agents and laxatives can be prescribed. The stool softeners bran, psyllium and docusates (up to 400 mg/day) are effective within 1–3 days
- Enemas may be effective in difficult cases.

Advanced Parkinson's Disease— Nonpharmacologic Approach to Associated Disorders

Swallowing Problems and Sialorrhea

These disorders may develop at any stage of PD and can be thoroughly evaluated by a speech therapist. Symptoms may include:
- Choking
- Coughing
- Drooling
- Holding.

Motor problems contributing to these difficulties include:
- Decreased tongue mobility
- Decreased elevation of the larynx
- Impaired swallowing reflex
- Diminished pharyngeal peristalsis.

Patients may fail to swallow saliva automatically resulting in poling in the mouth and throat. Saliva build up may also contribute to muffled speech. Careful attention to process of swallowing may help in improve sialorrhea and related problems. Patients should be advised to consciously swallow saliva frequently. Holding the head upright helps to prevent pooling and enhance the swallowing mechanism. Finally; a conscious effort to swallow saliva must be made before speaking.

They should eat slowly, taking only small amounts of food with each bite. Food should be chewed thoroughly and swallowed before the next bite is taken.

Dental Care

Number of medications, including anticholinergics and antidepressants, commonly prescribed for Parkinson's patients cause xerostomia by suppressing the production of saliva thus reducing its antibacterial and cleaning actions resulting in an increased risk for coronal and root surface caries, periodontal disease, and tongue erosion.

Denture retention depends to a large extent to appropriate muscle function. Tremors and dyskinesias affecting the tongue may dislodge a mandibular denture and rigid and uncontrolled facial muscles may prevent the maxillary denture from maintaining a good retentive seal.

The increased tendency to tooth decay in Parkinson's patient is now though to be the result of xerostomia and the decreased ability to perform regular oral hygiene. New varieties of electric and sonic toothbrushes facilitate dental care for Parkinson's patients. Dilute fluoride rinses, can be used daily as a 1-minute rinse to protect the teeth.

Nutritional Disturbances

Patients often have trouble preparing food, and eating or swallowing. In frustration, they may consume a very restricted diet, a problem enhanced by coexisting depression or dementia.

Specific dietary considerations for PD patients include:
- Patients with motor fluctuations may find that the medication is more effective if taken 30 minutes before meals
- Patients with severe fluctuations may eliminate protein during day to avoid this competition. All protein needs are then provided at the dinner.

Seborrheic Dermatitis

The cause of seborrheic demaititis and the reasons for its association with PD are unknown.

Although patients with PD tend to have long-term problems with seborrheic dermatitis, L-dopa tends to resolve the condition or decrease its severity.

The condition can usually be treated:
- Ketoconazole shampoo
- Shampoos and lotions containing selenium
- Shampoos, lotions, and creams containing pyrithione zinc.

Sexuality

In males, erectile dysfunction is most commonly described. Women it was found that women have anxiety, inhibition, and other concern.

In a recent open-label study, ten men had improved sexual function with the use of sildenafil 50 mg per encounter. No significant side effects were reported after eight encounters.

Levodopa may induce feelings of well-being and in some patients results in a significant but generally short-lied increase in sexually. Hypersexuality has also been described with dopaminergic therapy. Treatment of hyper sexuality includes counselling, lowering of the dose of medication and the possible use of an atypical antipsychotic agent.

Cardiopulmonary Impairment

- Patient's flexed posture can lead to kyphosis and cause a reduction in pulmonary capacity and restrictive lung disease pattern
- Breathing exercises, postural re-education and trunk exercises may be helpful
- Institute a general conditioning program to increase the patients' endurance
- If pulmonary function progressively worsens, assisted coughing techniques, incentive spirometry therapy intervention may be required.

Surgical Intervention

Surgical management of PD has been of increased interest over the past few years. Three main techniques currently in use include destructive therapy (lesioning) deep brain chronic stimulation, and transplantation.[9,10]
- Destructive therapy
- Lesioning options include thalamotomy is quite effective at relieving tremor, but its effects on the other clinical manifestations of PD seem to be less significant and more variable. Thalamotomy usually is reserved for a relatively small percentage of patients with predominantly drug-resistant tremor
- At present, palidotomy is the surgical procedure most commonly used for PD. Surgery employs lesioning to disrupt the abnormal activity in the globus pallidus to disinhibit the motor thalamus and cortical motor areas, ther by improving motor functioning. Candidates for palidotomy include patients who are disabled despite optimal medical management and who have responded to L-dopa therapy in the past but have developed complications from long-term L-dopa treatment. Rigidity, tremor and bradykinesia all seem to respond to palidotomy.

Deep Brain Stimulation[9,11]

- Chronic deep brain stimulation (DBS) seems to have emerged as an alternative to lesioning in patients with PD
- Stimulation has the advantages of safety, reversibility and adaptability (i.e., stimulation parameters can be adjusted as the clinical features change over time
- Stimulation sites include the ventral lateral thalamic nuclei (performed to

decrease tremor with a good response in 80–85% of patients), the globus pallidus (for bradykinesia, gait, speech, drug-induced dyskinesias), and the subthalamic nucleus (for bradykinesia, rigidity, tremor, gait/posture). A recent study of six male patients showed improved motor rating scores, reduced timing and spatial errors following DBS of the internal globus pallidus.

Transplantation

Although stimulation and lesioning can improve symptoms, neither corrects the underlying pathology of the disease, which is a lack of DA from loss of substantia nigra neurons. Transplantation therapy offers the possibility of replacing these lost neurons.[12]

- Clinical trials have examined the use of three types of transplants, autologous adrenal medulla transplants, fetal mesencephalon grafts, and xenografts
- Adrenal medulla transplants are not in widespread use because of the high morbidity and mortality from adrenalectomy
- Fetal mesencephalon grafts have shown promising early results. Trials continue, but ethical concerns, insufficient tissue, and procedural difficulties make it unlikely for the procedure to become common place
- The most common xenograft used is the fetal big mesencephalon. A trial currently is underway to determine the efficacy of this procedure.

Rehabilitation

Nonpharmacologic therapy, especially psychological support is of incalculable value from diagnosis throughout the course of PD. Patients derive benefits from the knowledge that the disease is an area of active research and the increasingly effective medications and other interventions are on the horizon.

The comprehensive management of PD patients is a team effort involving a variety of therapeutic interventions and therapists, include the:

- Primary physician
- Neurologist
- Family members
- Physical, occupational, and speech therapists.

Although the diagnosis and management plan of PD and related movement disorders are largely handled by neurologists, family or primary physicians. They are often the first to suspect the diagnosis and to refer patients to specialists and are likely to provide coordination of therapy thereafter.

Patient Education

Topics for discussion early in the course of Parkinson's disease:
- At Diagnosis
  - Outline general nature of Parkinson's disease and its treatability.
- 1–2 months
  - Explain prognosis of typical case
  - Outline ongoing research related to prophylaxis and treatment
  - Recommend patient education literature
  - Recommend joining national support societies
  - Follow-up, rereading, national support societies.
- 8 months
  - Educate regarding treatment complications to be aware of
  - Dose-related wearing off
  - Dyskinesia
  - Mental difficulty.
- 2 years
  - Recommend joining local support group
  - Recommend regular exercise schedule, if patient is sedentary.

Environmental Modifications

The first level of adaptation of PD revolves around the patient's environment, which should be evaluated during a home visit by an occupational therapist.

- A bed low enough to allow the patient to rise early
- A chair with arm rests and a firm seat to facilitate dressing
- A urinal or commode near the bed for nighttime use

- If stiffness is a problem a bed cradle made from a study cardboard box will keep bed clothes from entangling beet and lower leg when the patients turns in bed
- A trapeze over head of the bed or a cord attached to the frame may help in changing position or rising
- Button fasteners, zipper extensions, and elastic shoe laces.

Bathroom

- A raised toilet seat and a grab bar on the adjacent wall
- A toothpaste tube squeezer and a large handled tooth brush
- An elastic razor
- Pub and shower seats grab bars
- Soap on a rope, sponge on a long handle.

Kitchen

- Utensils with larger handles and knives that cut with rocking motion
- Combination utensils such as combined fork and spoon
- Easy hold cups, flexible plastic straws, and nonskid plates.

Daily Living

- A push button telephone adapted with larger keys
- A book holder to help stabilize pages.

Driving

- Considerations in assessing driving ability should include
- Judgment
- Mental status
- Reaction speed

The tendency to freeze can be fatal. Since the decision regarding driving is always difficult, the most objective approach is to have the patient take an approved driver instruction course or retake the state driver's license test.

Physical Therapy

Walking 1 mile a day is often considered to reasonable goal, although many patients can walk much further than that. Swimming is often recommended, especially for patients who swam earlier in life.

Patients who play golf, tennis, or racquet ball or those who hike, bicycle or jog should be encouraged to continue these activities on a regular basis

Back thigh stretches: This exercise is designed to reduce tightness and cramping in the back thigh muscles.

- *Position*: Lie on your back with your knees bent. Arms are stretched above your head.
- *Action:*
  - Raise your right knee
  - Stretch your-heel toward the ceiling
  - Point your toes toward your nose
  - Bend your right knee and place it back at the start position
  - Repeat, raising the right knee
  - Stretch your heel toward the ceiling
  - Point your toes towards your nose
  - Do ten stretches, alternating legs.

High Step Marching

Marching while walking is designed to challenge you to lift your feet with every step and also loosens the hips.
- *Action*: Bring your legs toes and knee up with every step you take. March as you walk.

Arm X's and Y's

This exercise is helpful for deep breathing and posture
- *Position:* Lie on your back. Your legs are straight, hands crossed and touching the upper thighs
- *Action*:
  - Spread your hands as you inhale and raise the arms over your head up and out to make a V
  - Make fists and exhale as you lower your arms across your hips making X
  - Rest and repeat ten times
  - At another time; sit in a straight chair with your wrists crossed on top of your knees
  - Perform this movement as above from the seated position
  - For more exertion small hand weights may be used to increase your strength.

Shift, Lift, and Step
Stand straight with feet 6 inches apart. Hands open arms at your sides. For extra safety stand in front of a chair.
- Action:
  - Shift your weight of you left leg as you lift your right toes and step forward on heel, then toes down. Balance and step back
  - Shift your right leg as you lift left toes and step toward as before
  - Balance and step back. Do ten times alternating legs.

Symptoms of slowness and stiffness may be improved by repetitive movement exercise.

Gait Disturbance
A focused approach to gait disorders involves, hesitation when starting to walk (start hesitation) and the temporary inability to move (freezing) can sometimes be overcome by issuing verbal commands (" ready, set, go").

Patients with postural inability may be walking with a few involuntary steps backward. Since these patients have a tendency to fall, their shoes should have leather not rubber, soles, and heel lifts to help tilt them forward.

Speech Therapy
A major source of disability in PD is disordered speech, hypophonia, dysarthria and reduced variability in pitch and rhythm. Poor respiratory, rigidity and bradykinesia involving the speech musculature aggravate all these problems.

Speech therapy emphasizes breathing control: patients practice augmentation of voice loudness and variation in pitch. Exercises are intended to increase the number of words spoken with each breath. Patients may also find that reading or singing aloud is a good practice exercise.

Occupational Therapy
Employment may be either the patient's usual premorbid occupation or a new type of work more appropriate for an individual with a movement disorder. Many PD patients are able to remain employed for a long time, often through making selective adaptations.

Recreational Therapy
Because of the high level of impairment and disability seen in many patients with PD. It is not surprising that vocational pursuits often become more difficult. This change certainly can have a detrimental impact on the patient's overall quality of life. A recreational therapist may be helpful in identifying previous recreational interest and in helping the patient to pursue them once more, with or without assistance. In case where this is not possible, new interests can be identified and explored. The therapeutic value of social and recreational pursuits should not be underestimated in these patients, as many can feel isolated and lonely because of the effects of the disease.

Psychotherapy and Counseling
The psychological changes that affect PD patients can be more devastating than the motor impairment particularly early in the disease. Moreover, emotional stress can increase motor symptoms. The most common psychological problem faced by the patients is depression. Refer patients and their families to a psychological counselor experienced with the mental and emotional problem of the disease.

Psychologists and social workers can be an important part of the healthcare team. Adjustment to a diagnosis of Parkinson disease is often stressful, and sometimes prolonged.

Overtime, people get past the feelings of being overwhelmed with the diagnosis, and begin to plan how to accommodate the reality of PD in their live. Short-term counseling with a capable psychotherapist can be immensely helpful during this period. In addition to responses, PD is sometimes accompanied by depression and anxiety. Dopamine, which is depleted in PD, is not the only neurotransmitter produced in the brain.

Other chemical messengers, such a serotonin, can also become out of balance, these neurotransmitters are involved in mood. Clinical depression can sometimes abate spontaneously, but prolonged depression wreaks havoc with energy levels, productivity, and close relationships. If you experience mood changes and low spirits for more than 2 weeks, ask your physician to refer you to a competent therapist. In addition, your doctor may prescribe an antidepressant medication that can safely be taken with anti-Parkinson's drugs.

Common family reactions include anger and concomitant guilt, fatigue, and social isolation. Helping the family or caregivers to understand PD. Family members or caregiver should be encouraged to accompany patients to physician.

Assessment Scales in Parkinson's Disease

Table 1: Unified Parkinson's Disease Rating Scale	
Mentation, behavior, and mood	
Intellectual impairment	
0	None
1	Mild consistent forgetfulness with partial recollection of event and no other difficulties
2	Moderate memory loss, with disorientation and moderate difficulty handling complex problems. Mild but definite impairment of function at home with a need of occasional prompting
3	Severe memory loss with disorientation for time and often for place. Severe impairment in handling problems
4	Severe memory loss with orientation preserved to person only. Unable to make judgment or solve problems. Requires much help with personal care. Cannot be left alone at all
Thought disorder (due to dementia or drug intoxication)	
0	None
1	Vivid dreaming
2	"Benign" hallucinations with insight retained
3	Occasional to frequent hallucination or delusions without insight could interfere with daily activities
4	Persistent hallucination, delusions, or florid psychosis. Not able to care for self

Continued

Continued

Depression	
0	Not present
1	Periods of sadness of guilt greater than normal, never sustained for days or weeks
2	Sustained depression (1 week or more)
3	Sustained depression with vegetative symptoms (insomnia, anorexia, weight loss, and loss of interest)
4	Sustained depression with vegetative symptoms and suicidal thoughts or intent
Motivation/initiative	
0	Normal
1	Less assertive than usual, more passive
2	Loss of initiative or disinterest in elective (nonroutine) activities
3	Loss of initiative or disinterest in day-to-day (routine) activities
4	Withdrawn, complete loss of motivation
Activities of daily living (determine for "on"/"off")	
Speech	
0	Normal
1	Mildly affected; no difficulty being understood
2	Moderately affected; sometimes asked to repeat statements
3	Severely affected; frequently asked to repeat statement
4	Unintelligible most of the time
Salivation	
0	Normal
1	Slight but definitive excess of saliva in mouth; may experience nighttime drooling
2	Moderately excessive saliva; may experience minimal drooling
3	Marked excess of saliva with some drooling
4	Marked drooling constantly requires tissue or handkerchief
Swallowing	
0	Normal
1	Rare choking

Continued

Continued

2	Occasional choking
3	Requires soft food
4	Requires nasogastric tube or gastrostomy feeding
Handwriting	
0	Normal
1	Slightly or small
2	Moderately slow or small; all words are legible
3	Severely affected; not all words are legible
4	The majority of words are not legible
Cutting food and handling utensils	
0	Normal
1	Somewhat slow and clumsy, but not help needed
2	Can cut most foods, although clumsy and slow; some help needed
3	Food must be cut by someone, but can still feed self slowly.
4	Needs to be fed
Dressing	
0	Normal
1	Somewhat slow, but not help needed
2	Occasional assistance with buttoning, getting arms in to sleeves
3	Considerable help required, but can do some things alone
4	Helpless
Hygiene	
0	Normal
1	Somewhat slow, but no help needed
2	Needs help to shower or bathe; very slowly in hygiene care
3	Requires assistance for washing, brushing teeth, combing hair, and use the toilet
4	Helpless (Foley catheter or other mechanical aids needed)
Turning in bed and adjusting bed clothes	
0	Normal
1	Somewhat slow and clumsy, but no help needed

Continued

2	Can turn alone or adjust sheets, but with great difficulty.
3	Can initiate movement, but not turn or adjust sheet alone
4	Helpless
Falling (Unrelated to freezing)	
0	None
1	Rare falling
2	Occasionally falls, less than once per day
3	Falls of an average of once daily
4	Falls more than once daily
Freezing when walking	
0	None
1	Rare freezing when walking; may have start hesitation
2	Occasional freezing when walking
3	Frequent freezing; occasionally falls due to freezing
4	Frequent falls due to freezing
Walking	
0	Normal
1	Mild difficulty; may not swing arms or may tend to drag leg
2	Moderate difficulty but requires little or no assistance
3	Cannot walk at all, even with assistance
Tremor	
0	Absent
1	Slight and infrequently present
2	Moderate; bothersome to patient
3	Severe; interferes with many activities
4	Marked; interferes with most activities
Sensory complaints related to Parkinsonism	
0	None
1	Occasionally has numbness, tingling, or mild aching
2	Frequently has numbness, tingling or aching; not distressing
3	Frequently painful sensations
4	Excruciating pain

Continued *Continued*

Continued

	Motor examination (determine for "on"/"off")
0	Normal
1	Slight loss of expression, diction, and/or volume
2	Monotone, slurred but understandable; moderately impaired
3	Marked impairment, difficult to understand
4	Unintelligible
	Facial expression
0	Normal
1	Slight hypomimia, could be normal "poker face"
2	Slight but definitely abnormal diminution of facial expression
3	Moderate hypomimia; lips parted some of the time
4	Masked or fixed facies with severe or complete loss of facial expression; lips parted one-fourth inch or more
	Tremor at rest
0	Absent
1	Slight and infrequent present
2	Mild in amplitude and persistent; or, moderate in amplitude but only intermittently present
3	Moderate in amplitude and present most of the time
4	Marked in amplitude and present most of the time
	Action of postural tremor of hands
0	Absent
1	Slight; present with action
2	Moderate in amplitude; present with action
3	Moderate in amplitude with posture holding as well a action
4	Marked in amplitude; interferes with feeding
	Rigidity (judged on passive movement of major joints with patient relaxed in sitting position. Cogwheeling to ignored)
0	Absent
1	Slight or detachable only when activated by mirror and other movements
2	Mild to moderate

Continued

3	Marked, but full range of motion easily achieved
4	Severe, range of motion achieved with difficulty
	Finger taps (patient taps thumb with index finger in rapid succession with widest amplitude possible, each hand separately)
0	Normal (>15/5 s)
1	Mild slowing and / or reduction in amplitude (11–14/5 s)
2	Moderately impaired. Definite early fatiguing. May have occasional arrests in movement (7–10/5 s)
3	Severely impaired. Frequent hesitation in initiating movements or arrests in movement (3–6/5 s)
4	Can barely perform the task (0–2/5 s)
	Hand movements (patient opens and closes hands in rapid succession with widest amplitude possible, each hand separately)
0	Normal
1	Mild slowing and/or reduction in amplitude
2	Moderately impaired. Definite and early fatiguing. May have occasional arrests in movement
3	Severely impaired. Frequent hesitation in initiating movements or arrests in ongoing movement
4	Can barely perform the task
	Rapid altering movements (pronation-supination movements of hands, vertically or horizontally, with as large an amplitude as possible, both hands simultaneously)
0	Normal
1	Mild slowing and/or reduction in amplitude
2	Moderately impaired. Definite and early fatiguing. May have occasional arrests in movement
3	Severely impaired. Frequent hesitation in initiating movements or arrests in ongoing movement
4	Can barely perform the task

Continued

Continued

Leg agility (with knee bent patient taps heel on ground in rapid succession, picking up entire leg. Amplitude should be about 3 inches)	
0	Normal
1	Moderately slowing and/or reduction in amplitude
2	Moderately impaired. Definite and early fatiguing. May have occasional arrests in movement
3	Severely impaired frequent hesitation in initiating movements or arrest in ongoing movement
4	Can barely perform the task
Rising from chair (patient attempts to arise from a straight-back wood or metal chair with arms folded across chest)	
0	Normal
1	Slow; or may need than one attempt
2	Pushes self-up from arms of seat
3	Tends to fall back and may have to try more than one time but can get up without help
4	Unable to rise without help
Posture	
0	Normal erect
1	Not quite erect, slightly stooped posture; could be normal for older person
2	Moderately stopped posture, definitely abnormal; can be slightly leaning to one side
3	Severely stooped posture with kyphosis; can be moderately leaning to one side
4	Marked flexion with extreme abnormality to posture
Gait	
0	Normal
1	Walks slowly, may shuffle with short steps, but no restination or propulsion
2	Walks with difficulty, but requires little or no assistance, may have some festination, short steps or propulsion
3	Severe disturbance of gait, requiring assistance
4	Cannot walk at all, even with assistance

Continued

Postural stability (response to sudden posterior displacement produced by pull or shoulders while patient is erect, with eyes open and feet slightly apart. Patient is prepared)	
0	Normal
1	Retropulsion, but recovers unaided
2	Absence of postural response; would fall if not caught by examiner
3	Very unstable, tends to lose balance spontaneously
4	Unstable to stand without assistance
Body bradykinesia and hypokinesia (combining slowness, hesitance, decreased arm swing, small amplitude, and poverty of movement in general)	
0	None
1	Minimal slowness, giving movements a deliberate character, could be normal for some persons. Possibly reduced amplitude.
2	Mild degree of slowness and poverty of movement that is definitely abnormal. Alternatively, some reduced amplitude
3	Moderate slowness, poverty or small amplitude of movement
4	Marked slowness, poverty or small amplitude of movement
Complications of therapy (with in the past week)	
Dyskinesias	
Duration: What proportion of the walking day are dyskinesias present? (historical information)	
0	None
1	1–25% of day
2	26–50% of day
3	51–75% of day
4	76–100% of day
Disability: How disabling are the dyskinesia? (historical information; may be modified by office)	
0	Not disabling
1	Mildly disabling
2	Moderately disabling
3	Severely disability
4	Completely disabled

Continued

Continued

Painful dyskinesia: How painful are the dyskinesia?	
0	No painful dyskinesia
1	Slight
2	Moderate
3	Severely disabling
4	Completely disabled
Presence of early morning dystonia (historical information)	
0	No
1	Yes
Clinical fluctuations	
Are any "off" periods predictable as to timing after a dose or medication?	
0	No
0	Yes
Are any "off" periods unpredictable as to timing after a dose or medication?	
0	No
1	Yes
Do any of the "off" periods come on suddenly (e.g., over a few seconds)?	
0	No
1	Yes
What proportions of the walking day is the patient "off" on average?	
0	None
1	1–25% of day
2	26–50% of day
3	51–75% of day
4	76–100% of day
Other complications	
Does the patients have anorexia, nausea, or vomiting?	
0	No
1	Yes
Does the patients have any sleep disturbance (e.g., insomnia or hypersomnolence)?	
0	No
1	Yes
Does the patient have symptomatic orthostasis?	
0	No
1	Yes

Table 2: Record the patient's blood pressure, pulse, and weight on the scoring form	
Part A: Modified Hoehn and Yahr Staging	
Stage 0	No signs of disease
Stage 1	Unilateral disease
Stage 1.5	Unilateral plus axial involvement
Stage 2	Bilateral disease, without impairment of balance
Stage 2.5	Mild bilateral disease, with recovery on pull test
Stage 3	Mild-to-moderate bilateral disease; some postural inability; physical independent
Part B: Schwab and England Activities of Daily Living Scale	
100%	Completely independent. Able to do all chores without slowness, difficulty, or impairment. Especially normal. Unaware of any difficulty
90%	Completely independent. Able to do all chores with some degree of slowness, difficulty, and impairment. Might take twice as long. Beginning to be aware of difficulty
80%	Completely independent in most chores. Takes twice as long. Conscious of difficulty and slowness
70%	Not completely independent. More difficulty with some chores than others. Takes 3 to 4 times as-long to complete some chores. Must spend a large part of the day with chores
60%	Not completely independent. Can do most chores, but exceedingly slowly and with much effort. Makes errors; some chores impossible
50%	More dependent. Help with half the chores lower etc. difficulty with everything
40%	Very dependent. Can assist with all chores, but can do few alone
30%	With effort, now and then does a few chores alone or begins alone. Much help needed
20%	Nothing alone. Can be a slight help with some chores. Severe invalid
10%	Totally dependent, helpless. Complete invalid
0%	Vegetative, functions such as swallowing, bladder and bowel functions are not functioning. Bedridden

REFERENCES

1. Jancovic J, The extra pyramidal disorders In: Bennet JC Plum F eds Cecil Text book of Medicine 20 Edition. Philadelphia, PA: WB Saunders Co. 1996: 2042-6.
2. Adams RD Victor, Principles of Neurology 7th Edition, New York, NY: McGrawHill: 2001: 1067-78.
3. Goldman SM Tanner. Etiology of Parkinson's disease. In: Jancovic J Tolosa E, eds Parkinson's Disease and Movement Disorder 3rd ed Baltimore Md: Lippincott Williams and Wilkins: 1998: 133-58.
4. Stoess JA. Etiology of Parkinson's disease. Can J Neurol Sci. 1992;26:Suppl 2:5-12.
5. Poewee WH, Wenning GK. The natural history of PD. Neurology. 1996:47:S146-52.
6. Golbe LI, Sage JI. Medical treatment of Parkinson's disease; In Kurlan R ed Treatment of Movement Disorders Philadephia, PA: JB Lippencott Co; 1995:1-56.
7. Waters CH. Neurology. 1997;(1-Suppl 1):S47-57.
8. Waters CH. Managing late complications of PD. Neurology. 1997;49:S49-57.
9. Lopiano I, Rizzone M, Bergamaco B, et al. Deep brain stimulation of the subthalamic nucleus in PD an analysis of the exclusion causes. J Neurol Sci. 2002;195(2):167-70.
10. Hallett M, Litvan I, the Task Force on Surgery for Surgery for Parkinon'sDiease. Evaluation of surgery for Parkinson's Disease. A report of the therapeutics and technology assessment sub committee of the American Academy of Neurology. Neurology. 1999;53;1910-21.
11. Schuurman PR, Bosch DA, Bosuyt PM, et al. A comparison of continuous thalamic stimulation and thalamotomy for suppression of severe tremor (see comments). N Engl J Med 2000;342(7):461-8.
12. Hallett M, Litvan I. Evaluation of surgery for Parkinson's disease: A report of the therapeutics and technology Assessment Subcommittee of the American Academy of Neurology. The Task Force on surgery for Parkinson's Disease. Neurology. 1999;53(9):1910-21.

CHAPTER 10

Neurological Manifestations of Thyroid Disorders

Adhiti Krishnamoorthy

INTRODUCTION

Thyroid disease is one of the most frequently encountered problems in outpatient clinics. The spectrum of presenting may extend from vague presentations with fatigue, disturbances in appetite and nonspecific aches and pains to characteristic clinical features described in hyperthyroidism (symptoms: heat intolerance, palpitations, tremors, increased sweating, anxiety, restlessness, irritability, loss of weight despite an increased appetite; signs: clubbing, resting tachycardia, exophthalmos, pretibial myxedema, goiter, thyroid bruit) and hypothyroidism (symptoms: cold intolerance, lethargy, mental dullness, cognitive slowing, hoarseness of voice, weight gain despite increase in appetite, menstrual disturbances; signs: coarse and dry skin, apathy, bradycardia, delayed relaxation of deep tendon reflexes, goiter). The neurological manifestations described in thyroid dysfunction are varied and may even be the first presentation of the thyroid disease. Therefore, in patients presenting with these problems, the possibility of an underlying thyroid disorder needs to be considered.

The neurological manifestations of thyroid disorders can be grouped into:
- Manifestations arising from thyroid hormone imbalance (excess/deficiency)
- Manifestations arising from shared etiological factors (like autoimmune basis or genetic susceptibility).

NEUROLOGICAL MANIFESTATIONS RELATED TO THYROID HORMONE IMBALANCE

These manifestations directly result from a state of thyroid hormone excess or deficiency and hence, are partly or completely responsive to treatment of the underlying hypo or hyperthyroid state. The intensity of clinical features may be directly related to the duration or severity of thyroid dysfunction.

Neurological Manifestations of Hyperthyroidism

Cognitive Impairment

This is common in patients with hyperthyroidism, especially in elderly. The spectrum of manifestations varies from mild confusion to frank dementia. Cognitive impairments are seen commonly in the form of impaired attention, orientation, and immediate recall. Behavioral and personality changes are also frequently encountered and may include anxiety, restlessness, emotional lability, and rarely agitation and psychosis.[1] In the elderly, a less active form called "apathetic thyrotoxicosis" has also been described, characterized predominantly by depression and lethargy. Dementia and confusion were observed in 33% and 18% respectively of elderly patients with thyrotoxicosis.[2] Even in younger patients with subclinical hyperthyroidism, their cognitive scores were found to be much lower than their euthyroid counterparts.[3] The onset is often subacute, although it may be fulminant in thyroid storm, progressing through delirium to somnolence and coma.[4] These features have not been associated with specific abnormalities on imaging or electroencephalography (EEG). Treatment of the hyperthyroid state results in improvement of inattention and frontal lobe impairment although there may be residual cognitive impairment.

Seizures

Seizures may be encountered in the encephalopathy seen with acute thyrotoxicosis. They may be focal or generalized and are usually accompanied by hyper-reflexia and tremors.[5] They are more commonly experienced in thyroid storm, and on occasions with status epilepticus.[6] Even the EEG abnormalities (which are most often nonspecific) are found to reverse with thyroid lowering treatment in individual cases.

Cerebrovascular Accidents

It has been observed that cerebrovascular accidents, especially ischemic strokes, occur more commonly in hyperthyroid patients.[7] The most common cause of stroke in hyperthyroidism is atrial fibrillation-associated embolic phenomena. Although atrial fibrillation is seen in 10-15% of hyperthyroid patients, hyperthyroidism per se contributes to only one percent (or lesser) cases of atrial fibrillation. Cortical venous thrombosis (CVT) have also been associated with strokes in hyperthyroid patients. Hyperthyroidism is thought to result in a hypercoagulable state which is in turn responsible for CVTs.[8]

Movement Disorders

Tremors are one of the better described clinical features consistently affiliated with hyperthyroidism. They are seen in up to 76% of such patients.[9] The fine tremors of hyperthyroidism are characterized by high frequency and low amplitude, very similar to essential tremors. The key differentiating feature lies in the responsiveness of the former to beta blockers. Chorea (especially involving the extremities) and rarely myoclonus and ballism have also been reported in patients with hyperthyroidism.[10]

Thyrotoxic Periodic Paralysis

This pure motor syndrome presents with symmetric ascending acute flaccid paralysis. This has been most reported from males of Asian origin in the age groups of 20-40 years.[11] Common precipitants include heavy carbohydrate load, high salt diet, alcohol, excessive exercise, infection, and use of beta-agonists. Clinical examination may reveal proximal predominant weakness. Deep tendon reflexes are diminished or even absent in the majority. Ocular, bulbar, and respiratory involvement is unusual. The attack is usually preceded by a prodrome of muscle aches, stiffness, and cramps. Attacks usually occur in early mornings and in warm seasons. Investigations commonly reveal low serum potassium with low urinary potassium excretion rate and normal acid base balance. Low serum magnesium and phosphate levels are also common. A high urinary Ca/P ratio helps in distinguishing thyrotoxic periodic paralysis from the hereditary hypokalemic periodic paralysis. An increased Na^+/K^+-ATPase activity resulting directly from thyroid hormone excess and indirectly from the hyperadrenergic state (and hyperinsulinemia) has been traditionally thought to be the culprit; but, more recently, loss of function mutations in the Kir2.6 potassium channel and single nucleotide polymorphisms in the Cav1.1 calcium channel have been implicated. Electrocardiography abnormalities include sinus tachycardia, high voltage QRS and first degree atrioventricular block. Electromyography reveals reduced CMAP (compound muscle action potential) and nerve conduction velocity studies are normal. The importance of differentiating this from the hereditary hypokalemic periodic paralysis lies in management, as the former requires beta blockade in addition to potassium correction (the dose of which is also significantly reduced by beta blockers). Excessive potassium correction (>20 mEq/hour) may result in rebound hyperkalemia during the recovery of paralysis. Although potassium supplements have no role in the prophylaxis, oral non selective beta-blockers play an important role in preventing and ameliorating further recurrences.[12]

Myopathy

The muscle weakness associated with hyperthyroidism has been seen in 60–80% of patients and has been commonly described in patients above the age of 40 years.[9] The risk of myopathy is proportional to the duration of the disease. It may be acute or chronic. The acute form has been seen in severe thyrotoxicosis and it involves proximal and distal and rarely bulbar and respiratory muscles.[13] Rhabdomyolysis has also been seen in this scenario. The chronic form has a subacute onset (weeks to months after onset of hyperthyroidism) and has been described in patients with long standing hyperthyroidism. It involves primarily the proximal groups of muscles, especially the hip flexors and the knee extensors. Rarely orbital myositis has been described that manifests as weakness and pain in the extraocular muscles. In hyperthyroid myopathy, muscle cramps, atrophy, and elevations in creatine kinase (CK) levels are less common.[9] Electromyography may be normal or may show a typical myopathic pattern in the more proximal groups of muscles. Beta-blockade in conjunction with antithyroid drugs largely help in recovering the muscle function.

Peripheral Neuropathy

Distal sensory predominant axonal neuropathy has been often described in (nearly 20%) hyperthyroid patients. Weakness evolves early in the course of the disease and resolves rapidly with treatment. Carpal tunnel syndrome has been described in 5–7% of hyperthyroid patients,[9] and rarely trigger finger and Dupuytren's contractures have also been reported to be more prevalent.[14] There have also been reports of a polyneuropathy presenting with acute areflexic quadriparesis, with the lower limbs more severely affected, in the setting of severe thyrotoxicosis or thyroid storm. This has also been referred to as Basedow's paraparesis.[15]

Note on Management of Hyperthyroidism

The management of hyperthyroidism includes addressing the symptoms (beta-blockers) and the thyroid hormone excess (antithyroid drugs). Antithyroid drugs largely belong to the class of thionamides (propylthiouracil, methimazole, and carbimazole) form the cornerstone of medical management of thyrotoxicosis. They inhibit organification and coupling and hence the synthesis and release of thyroid hormone. It takes 2–8 weeks for a reduction in thyroid hormone synthesis to become clinically evident and hence beta blockers play a vital role in offering symptom control in this interval. As methimazole is more potent and longer acting (with once daily dosing) than propylthiouracil, it is preferred in most situations except the first trimester of pregnancy (methimazole and carbimazole are associated with teratogenesis) and thyroid storm (propylthiouracil has the additional effect of inhibiting the peripheral conversion of T4 to T3), where the latter is considered the agent of choice. The general principles of managing thyrotoxicosis include:

- Start the patient on low dose of antithyroid medications
    - Propylthiouracil (start with 50 mg BD/TID—can go up to 100–200 mg BD/TID) (max: 600 mg/day)
    - Methimazole (start with 5 mg OD—can go up to 30 mg/day)
    - Carbimazole (start with 5 mg OD—can go up to 40 mg/day).
- Add a beta-blocker for control of hyperadrenergic symptoms and to tide over the latent period
    - Propranolol (also inhibits peripheral conversion of T4 to T3) (10–20 mg TID/QID)
    - Atenolol (25–50 mg OD).
- After initiation of antithyroid medications, monitor thyroid function tests on a monthly basis and optimize the dose further

- They should be monitored for allergic reactions (fever, rash, joint pains) and more serious adverse effects (agranulocytosis, hepatitis, polyarthritis, lupus like vasculitis), in the event of which these drugs need to be withheld
- Saturated solution of potassium iodide (1–2 drops twice a day for 2 weeks) helps in preoperative preparation and rapidly results in a near euthyroid state in conjunction with other medications
- Cholestyramine has also found to be effective in reducing the circulating thyroid hormone levels by decreasing the enterohepatic circulation (4 g TID for 4 weeks)
- Steroids are effective in management of thyroid ophthalmopathy (oral or even parenteral in severe cases) and dermopathy (topical).

Radio iodine ablation is a preferred mode of treatment in Grave's disease, especially in patients with intolerance to thionamides and in those with severe thyrotoxicosis. It is administered as a single oral dose and has very few adverse effects (hypothyroidism). It is contraindicated in pregnancy, lactation, children under 5 years of age and in those with severe ophthalmopathy (as it has been found to worsen the same – post radio ablation steroids for two months is found to be helpful).

After the advent of radio iodine ablation, the role of surgery is largely limited to those with intolerance, concerns, or contraindications to radio iodine therapy and those with very large goiters.

Sequelae of Fetal and Neonatal Hypothyroidism—Cretinism

The presence of maternal hypothyroidism in the first trimester confers the most risk to the development of fetal hypothyroidism, which eventually results in cretinism. Neonatal hypothyroidism is often the result of iodine deficiency and has a better prognosis.[16] Characteristic clinical features include microcephaly, coarse cry, blepharospasm, strabismus, sensorineural hearing loss, speech impairment, macroglossia, thickened subcutaneous tissue, hypotonia, pot-belly, umbilical hernia, persistent primitive reflexes, polyneuropathy, and myopathic weakness. Apathy, sleepiness, and mental dullness are also frequently observed. Thyroid dysgenesis and dyshormonogenesis contribute to 85% and 15% respectively of the cases of permanent congenital hypothyroidism. Neurocognitive outcomes can be optimized and normal growth and development may be ensured if levothyroxine is started at the earliest (preferably within the first 2 weeks of life).[17]

Neurological Manifestations of Hypothyroidism

Myxedema Coma

Severe hypothyroidism with physiological compromise results in this rare medical emergency. It is usually seen in patients with long standing undiagnosed hypothyroidism and is often precipitated by infection, surgery, trauma, drugs, or heart failure. It is characterized by hypothermia (resulting from reduced basal metabolic rate and oxygen consumption), hypoventilation (resulting from central depression of the respiratory drive and decreased responsiveness to hypoxic and hypercapnic stimuli), hypotension (resulting from decreased cardiac contractility and hence decreased stroke volume, and bradycardia), hyponatremia (resulting from decreased water excretion and increased antidiuretic hormone) and altered mental status (resulting from decreased cerebral perfusion, glucose utilization and oxygen consumption) that may range from confusion to coma. The most common causes of death are respiratory failure, sepsis, and gastrointestinal bleeding. Electrocardiography may show bradycardia, low amplitude administration of levothyroxine (T4 – 300–600 mcg IV stat followed by 50–100 mcg/day) and liothyronine (T3 – 5–20 mcg IV stat followed by 2.5–10 mcg IV q8h), parenteral corticosteroids and supportive measures (like rewarming, correction of hypoglycemia and hyponatremia).

Cognitive Impairment and Dementia

This is more common in hypothyroidism than hyperthyroidism. Nearly two-thirds of patients with overt hypothyroidism have impairment in attention and executive functions and generalized cognitive slowing.[18] There needs to be a lower threshold for treating subclinical hypothyroidism in patients with cognitive decline [thyroid stimulating hormone (TSH) >7]. Rarely, a syndrome of psychosis has been described in patients with overt hypothyroidism, which was earlier recognized by the term "myxedema madness". Headaches have also been reported at a greater frequency in patients with hypothyroidism. Clinical features seen in nondemented older adults include impairments in learning, visuo-spatial abilities, visual scanning, word fluency, attention, and motor speed. These defects improve significantly with thyroid hormone replacement.[19]

Movement Disorders

The clinical features of parkinsonism and hypothyroidism are quite similar and may often be confused. One may even mask the presence of the other condition, thereby resulting in delay in diagnosis. Levodopa can cause decrease in thyrotropin-releasing hormone (TRH) and hence in TSH levels. Therefore, in patients on levodopa treatment for parkinsonism, blood samples for thyroid evaluation need to be drawn at least 6–8 hours after the last levodopa dose to prevent false negative results.[20]

Hypothyroid Myopathy

Muscle fatigue, weakness, stiffness, myalgias, or cramps may be one of the presenting features of hypothyroidism. This is more common among females. Motor movements have reduced velocity with delayed relaxation of deep tendon reflexes. In myopathies associated with hypothyroidism, the CK levels are usually elevated (although it does not correlate with the severity of involvement) in contrast to the hyperthyroid myopathies, where they have been found to be normal.[21] The most common presentation is akin to polymyositis with proximal weakness and elevated CK. Sometimes, it may present with muscle enlargement (pseudohypertrophy) and stiffness. This condition has been recognized as Hoffman's syndrome. In children, a rare syndrome of proximal weakness with diffuse muscle enlargement has been described (Kocher–Debre–Semelaigne syndrome). Electromyography helps in differentiating the delayed muscle relaxation from myotonia. Muscle biopsy shows nonspecific type II muscle fiber atrophy. The muscle strength returns to near normal state on treatment of the hypothyroidism.[22]

Carpal Tunnel Syndrome

The most common form of peripheral neuropathy seen in patients with hypothyroidism is carpal tunnel syndrome, which is an entrapment neuropathy caused by compression of the median nerve at the carpal tunnel. Although carpal tunnel syndrome (CTS) is seen in nearly one-third of patients with hypothyroidism (29% in one study), hypothyroidism per se has been found to be responsible for only 1–10% of cases of CTS.[9] Increased body mass index is an important risk factor in the development of CTS in hypothyroidism. Most of the neuropathies improve within 3–6 months of treatment.[23]

Polyneuropathy

Hypothyroidism has been associated with a symmetric distal predominant sensorimotor axonal polyneuropathy, which is seen in nearly 40% of the former. Patients often complain of painful paresthesias. It involves the lower limbs more frequently than the upper limbs with a stocking and glove pattern. Deep tendon reflexes show delayed relaxation.[9]

Note on Management of Hypothyroidism

The management of hypothyroidism includes initiation of replacement doses of levothyroxine (1.6 mcg/kg/day). Most cases of mild-to-moderate hypothyroidism can be started on 50–75 mcg/day. They need to be followed on a 6–8 weekly basis and the dose should be titrated upwards (by 12.5–25 mcg/day) till target TSH is reached.

Clinical improvement occurs in a week while biochemical improvement takes 4–6 weeks on optimal dose. In patients with primary hypothyroidism, TSH serves as a marker of adequacy of treatment, while in those with secondary hypothyroidism, T4 serves the same purpose.

In patients with subclinical hypothyroidism, a TSH cut off of 10 has been assigned to initiate treatment (for values between 5 and 10, options need to be individualized and patients need to be closely monitored). In patients with elderly and those with ischemic heart disease, the starting dose is one-fourth of that which is recommended for their weight. In pregnancy and lactation, there is a lower threshold to treat subclinical hypothyroidism.

Neurological Manifestations Observed due to Shared Etiological Factors

These features arise mostly from the shared autoimmune etiology or less frequently, from the common genetic susceptibility loci. They may not be related to the onset of thyroid dysfunction (may precede or follow or occur concurrently) and hence may even be observed in euthyroid patients. These features respond to immunosuppression.

Myasthenia Gravis

Myasthenia gravis (MG) is a rare autoimmune condition characterized by autoantibody mediated injury to the neuromuscular junctions, resulting in blockade of synaptic transmission and hence fatigable symptomatic muscle weakness. The prevalence of hyperthyroidism has been found to be as high as 17% in patients with MG.[24] Myasthenia gravis has been found to coexist with a number of autoimmune diseases, the most common of which has been observed to be autoimmune thyroid disease (AITD) (which encompasses hyperthyroid patients with Grave's disease, hypothyroid patients with autoimmune thyroiditis and euthyroid patients with elevated titres of anti-thyroid antibodies). The HLA-DQ3 plays an important role in the pathogenesis.[25] Although AITD is more common among females, the occurrence of MG with AITD has been found to occur predominantly in males. Myasthenia gravis patients with AITD have been found to have a milder clinical expression, preferential ocular involvement and a lower frequency of thymic disease and acetylcholine receptor antibodies.[26]

Hashimotos Encephalopathy (Steroid Responsive Encephalopathy Associated with Autoimmune Thyroiditis)

A nonvasculitic autoimmune inflammatory meningoencephalitis has been described in association with autoimmune thyroiditis. This common in females and has been commonly observed in the fourth decade of life. It is has been described as a syndrome of subacute onset of altered sensorium, seizures, and myoclonus, that is associated with elevated levels of anti-thyroid antibodies and highly responsive to steroids. It is thought to result from an antibody or an immune complex mediated neuronal injury.[27] The presentation may be stroke-like, with subacute onset of multiple/recurrent episodes of focal deficits or altered sensorium; or dementia-like with slow progressive cognitive impairment. Neuropsychiatric disturbances have been frequently observed. There is no specific temporal association with the onset of thyroiditis. Most patients described were euthyroid at the time of presentation. Cerebrospinal fluid may show elevated protein and lymphocytic pleocytosis. Electroencephalography shows nonspecific abnormalities. Imaging is usually normal. Some cases have been reported to have hyperintensities in the subcortical white matter and hippocampi. Relapse may occur although residual cognitive deficits are less common. Although, steroids form the cornerstone of management, refractory cases and those with frequent relapses have been found to benefit from intravenous immunoglobulins, plasmapheresis, and immunosuppressants like cyclophosphamide and azathioprine.[28]

Acute and Chronic Inflammatory Demyelinating Polyneuropathy

Acute inflammatory demyelinating polyneuropathy (AIDP) and chronic inflammatory demyelinating polyneuropathy (CIDP) have been observed in patients with AITD, with patients presenting with flaccid ascending areflexic weakness (proximal predominant).[29,30]

Vasculopathy

In patients with AITD (especially Grave's), carotid dissection has been rarely described. This has been attributed to segmental mediolytic arteriopathy that has been noted in autopsy findings.[31,32] Some patients have also been reported to have stenoses of intracranial vessels giving a radiological appearance similar to Moya Moya disease.[31]

Vasculitides

Takayasu arteritis, giant cell arteritis and antiphospholipid syndrome have been described more often in patients with AITD.[33,34]

Note on Thyroid Associated Orbitopathy and Eye Signs

Thyroid-associated orbitopathy (TAO), also commonly referred by the term "Graves" ophthalmopathy may precede, coincide, or follow symptoms of dysthyroidism (80% comprised of hyperthyroids of Grave's and 20% comprised of euthyroids, Hashimoto's, thyroid malignancy and neck irradiation). It is characterized by lid retraction, proptosis, chemosis, periorbital edema, and altered ocular mobility. The pathophysiology can be explained by an autoantibody mediated lymphocytic infiltration and fibroblast modulation in the orbital tissue. Although it has a self-limiting course, there may be exacerbations. Symptoms may include redness, dryness, or puffiness of eyes, diplopia, visual or field loss and ocular pain. Several signs have been described (Table1). Thyroid-associated orbitopathy is the most common cause of unilateral or bilateral ptosis in adults. Both ptosis and pseudoptosis (when the opposite eye has retraction) are seen in TAO. Keratoconjunctivitis and conjunctival injection may complicate the picture. The inferior and then, the medial recti are the most commonly involved and hence patients may present with hypotropia or esotropia. Compressive optic neuropathy, choroidal folds, glaucoma, pretibial myxedema, and thyroid acropachy may accompany TAO. Steroids and smoking cessation play an important role in the management. Exposure keratitis needs to be identified and addressed. High-dose intravenous steroids are reserved for compressive optic neuropathy. In severe cases that worsen despite medical management, surgery and radiation may be considered. Radiation therapy is most effective when combined with steroids and if initiated within 7 months of onset. Post-treatment with steroids for 2 months has been shown to reduce the risk of exacerbation following Iodine $_{131}$ therapy.[35]

Table 1: Named eye signs in thyroid associated orbitopathy

Name of the sign	Description
Vigouroux	Eyelid fullness
Stellwag	Infrequent blinking resulting in "staring look"
Dalrymple	Upper lid retraction with scleral show
Mobius	Poor convergence
Von Graefe	Lid lag on down gaze
Joffroy	Absent creases in forehead on upper gaze
Ballet	Restriction in the movement of one or more extra ocular muscles
Grove	Resistance to pulling down the retracted upper lid
Rosenbach	Fine tremor in the upper lid
Jelink	Hyperpigmentation of the eyelid

CONCLUSION

The neurological manifestations of thyroid disease can involve any part of the neuraxis and may be the first presenting symptom; which necessitates a high degree of clinical suspicion and a keen eye to detail while examining a patient with a neurological condition. The manifestations (like cognitive impairment, myopathy, neuropathy) that directly arise from a state of thyroid hormone imbalance respond well to management of the latter. Autoimmune thyroid disease is associated with manifestations like myasthenia gravis, steroid responsive encephalopathy, demyelinating polyneuropathies, etc. that respond to immunosuppression.

REFERENCES

1. Stern RA, Robinson B, Thorner AR, et al. A survey study of neuropsychiatric complaints in patients with GravesAPHY to management of the latClin Neurosci. 1996;8(2):181-5.
2. Martin FI, Deam DR. Hyperthyroidism in elderly hospitalised patients. Clinical features and treatment outcomes. Med J Aust. 1996;164(4):200-3.
3. Wu T, Flowers JW, Tudiver F, et al. Subclinical thyroid disorders and cognitive performance among adolescents in the United States. BMC Pediatr. 2006;6:12.
4. Trasciatti S, Prete C, Palummeri E, et al. Thyroid storm as precipitating factor in onset of coma in an elderly woman: Case report and literature review. Aging Clin Exp Res. 2004;16(6):490-4.
5. Jabbari B, Huott AD. Seizures in thyrotoxicosis. Epilepsia. 1980;21(1):91-6.
6. Safe AF, Griffiths KD, Maxwell RT. Thyrotoxic crisis presenting as status epilepticus. Postgrad Med J. 1990;66(772):150-2.
7. Sheu JJ, Kang JH, Lin H-C, et al. Hyperthyroidism and risk of ischemic stroke in young adults: A 5-year follow-up study. Stroke. 2010;41(5):961-6.
8. Verberne HJ, Fliers E, Prummel MF, et al. Thyrotoxicosis as a predisposing factor for cerebral venous thrombosis. Thyroid Off J Am Thyroid Assoc. 2000;10(7):607-10.
9. Duyff RF, Van den Bosch J, Laman DM, van Loon BJ, Linssen WH. Neuromuscular findings in thyroid dysfunction: A prospective clinical and electrodiagnostic study. J Neurol Neurosurg Psychiatry. 2000;68(6):750-5.
10. Puri V, Chaudhry N. Paroxysmal kinesigenic dyskinesia manifestation of hyperthyroidism. Neurol India. 2004;52(1):10210204
11. Sonkar SK, Kumar S, Singh NK. Thyrotoxic hypokalemic periodic paralysis. Indian J Crit Care Med 2018;22(5):378-80.
12. Salih M, van Kinschot CMJ, Peeters RP, et al. Thyrotoxic periodic paralysis: An unusual presentation of hyperthyroidism. Neth J Med. 2017;75(8):315-20.
13. Couillard P, Wijdicks EFM. Flaccid quadriplegia due to thyrotoxic myopathy. Neurocrit Care. 2014;20(2):296-7.
14. Cakir M, Samanci N, Balci N, et al. Musculoskeletal manifestations in patients with thyroid disease. Clin Endocrinol (Oxf). 2003;59(2):162-7.
15. Pandit L, Shankar SK, Gayathri N, et al. Acute thyrotoxic neuropathy—Basedowat paraplegia revisited. J Neurol Sci. 1998;155(2):211-4.
16. Cao XY, Jiang XM, Dou ZH, et al. Timing of vulnerability of the brain to iodine deficiency in endemic cretinism. N Engl J Med. 1994;331(26):1739-44.
17. Leung AKC, Leung AAC. Evaluation and management of the child with hypothyroidism. Recent Pat Endocr Metab Immune Drug Discov. 2018.
18. Constant EL, Adam S, Seron X, et al. Anxiety and depression, attention, and executive functions in hypothyroidism. J Int Neuropsychol Soc JINS. 2005;11(5):535-44.
19. Osterweil D, Syndulko K, Cohen SN, et al. Cognitive function in non-demented older adults with hypothyroidism. J Am Geriatr Soc. 1992;40(4):325-35.
20. Munhoz RP, Teive HAG, Troiano AR, et al. ParkinsonzaLeiva MHB, Graff Hid dysfunction. Parkinsonism Relat Disord. 2004;10(6):381-3.
21. Sindoni A, Rodolico C, Pappalardo MA, et al. Hypothyroid myopathy: A peculiar clinical presentation of thyroid failure. Review of the literature. Rev Endocr Metab Disord. 2016;17(4):499-519.
22. Mastaglia FL, Ojeda VJ, Sarnat HB, et al. Myopathies associated with hypothyroidism: A review based upon 13 cases. Aust N Z J Med. 1988;18(6):799-806.
23. Karne SS, Bhalerao NS. Carpal tunnel syndrome in hypothyroidism. J Clin Diagn Res. 2016;10(2):OC36-38.
24. Ratanakorn D, Vejjajiva A. Long-term follow-up of myasthenia gravis patients with hyperthyroidism. Acta Neurol Scand. 2002;106(2):93-8.
25. Sekiguchi Y, Hara Y, Takahashi M, et al. Reverse , Takaha" relationship between Graves' disease and myasthenia gravis; clinical and immunological studies. J Med Dent Sci. 2005;52(1):43-50.
26. Marinn M, Ricciardi R, Pinchera A, et al. Mild clinical expression of myasthenia gravis associated with autoimmune thyroid diseases. J Clin Endocrinol Metab. 1997;82(2):438-43.
27. Menon V, Subramanian K, Thamizh JS. Psychiatric presentations heralding Hashimotons encephalopathy: A systematic review and analysis of cases reported in literature. J Neurosci Rural Pract. 2017;8(2):261-7.
28. Mocellin R, Walterfang M, Velakoulis D. Hashimoto Hashimotomoto Ha: Epidemiology, pathogenesis and management. CNS Drugs. 2007;21(10):799-811.

29. Kohli RS, Bleibel W, Bleibel H. Concurrent immune thrombocytopenic purpura and Guillain-Barre syndrome in a patient with Hashimoto's thyroiditis. Am J Hematol. 2007;82(4):307-8.
30. Polizzi A, Ruggieri M, Vecchio I, et al. Autoimmune thyroiditis and acquired demyelinating polyradiculoneuropathy. Clin Neurol Neurosurg. 2001;103(3):151-4.
31. Squizzato A, Gerdes VEA, Brandjes DPM, et al. Thyroid diseases and cerebrovascular disease. Stroke. 2005;36(10):2302-10.
32. Pezzini A, Del Zotto E, Mazziotti G, et al. Thyroid autoimmunity and spontaneous cervical artery dissection. Stroke. 2006;37(9):2375-7.
33. Hofbauer LC, Spitzweg C, Heufelder AE. Graves E. Gravesaves. Gravesraves. G primary antiphospholipid syndrome. J Rheumatol. 1996;23(8):1435-7.
34. Thomas RD, Croft DN. Thyrotoxicosis and giant-cell arteritis. Br Med J. 1974;2(5916):408-9.
35. Bahn RS. Gravesavophthalmopathy. N Engl J Med. 2010;362(8):726-38.

CHAPTER 11

Stroke and Motor Recovery

Ken Richter, Pratik Bhattacharya, Ramesh Madhavan

INTRODUCTION

Fifteen percent (one billion) of the global population experience disability due to different reasons, with the prevalence higher in developing countries. As the fifth common cause for mortality in the world, stroke is a leading cause of disability in the USA with about 3% of males and 2% of females affected.[1] It's a well-known fact that when the blood flow to the brain is reduced, ischemia to the brain causes core infarct with evidence based therapies including thrombolytics and mechanical thrombectomies helping in only salvaging the penumbra. Neuroprotection and stem cell therapies are still experimental with no large positive trials yet in the pipeline for recovery of the brain tissue. That said, many medications have been tried to promote motor recovery after stroke. In this section we will discuss three medication groups: serotonin reuptake inhibitors (SSRI), dopaminergic therapy with levodopa (L-dopa) and amphetamines and the data evaluating their use following stroke. In summary, the authors will give a practical overview about motor recovery after stroke, with questions and the best evidence, focusing especially on the different modes of therapies.

HOW DOES WEAKNESS IMPROVE DURING THE RECOVERY PHASE AFTER STROKE?

The mechanism is called neural plasticity, where activation and modulation of the neural networks of the ipsilateral and contralateral motor areas reorganize and maximize motor improvement.[2]

WHEN DO WE START REHABILITATION IN STROKE PATIENTS?

Rehabilitation of stroke remains a mystery to many physicians and clinicians. It has been referred to as a "black box".[3] The problem is that much of what we do does not have rigorous evidentiary support, although certainly there is clinical support for its effectiveness. We will attempt to summarize the key points. There is good evidence that stroke rehabilitation should start early.[4] However, there is a caveat here. High-dose, very early mobilization within 24 hours may actually worsen outcome at 3 months, but there does not seem to be any reason to rehabilitate a stable patient after that. A strong, compelling argument for the intensity of stroke rehabilitation comes from the literature supporting improved outcomes from inpatient rehab facilities compared with subacute rehabilitation.[4]

WHAT IS THE BEST THERAPEUTIC TRADITIONAL PHYSICAL APPROACH FOR TREATING STROKE PATIENTS?

There are neurodevelopmental therapy/ Bobath, the Brunnstrom method, as well as proprioceptive neuromuscular facilitation among others. None of them were shown to be superior in retrospective comparisons. So, with the present state of knowledge it is obvious that patients need to be in therapy, but there are multiple options for delivering this therapy. While the various approaches have ardent supporters, no one approach has risen to the top as the premier technique.

While there may be questions about what is the best therapy approach, there is no question that the amount of exercise is important. Exercise physiology shows that intense practice can influence neuromuscular changes. Just as with a medication, various "dosages" will have various physiologic effects, so will the dosage of therapy. Interesting work done at the Rehabilitation Institute of Chicago at Northwestern has shown that much of the success of many interventions utilized in patients post stroke may be the result of increasing intensity or dose.[5] For example, in walking studies, a focused stepping training that has high doses, such as 1500–4000 steps in a 1-hour session, may provide superior outcomes. It needs to be specific training that is focused towards the desired activity, so-called specificity of training. There seems to be a relationship between the amount of practice and improvements in walking outcomes post stroke.[6] Training improves daily stepping activity and gait efficiencies in individuals post stroke who have reached a "plateau" recovery.[6] The high-intensity training likely increases synaptic efficiency. Their ability in step training enhances locomotor recovery after spinal cord injury.[7] In doing the therapy, there are various goals. One of the goals is towards motor compensation. This is just to get the task done no matter what the neurologic pattern of movement. Another is working on trying to restore a normal movement pattern (i.e., to work towards recovery of the normal pattern.

Constraint-induced movement therapy (CIMT) is a technique that shows significant benefit. When there is an injury to the brain, we compensate, and the easiest way to do something is often used. This can result in a learned neglect. Constraint-induced movement therapy is used to prevent this neglect. The uninvolved extremity is restrained with either a sling or a glove to remind the patient to use the involved side. Now, to be effective, there must be some isolated motion on the paretic side with at least some voluntary wrist and finger extension. In its original form, CIMT was used for 3–6 hours a day for 5 days a week. There is a modified version that uses it 1 hour a day for 3 days a week for 10 days. The latter seems to be quite beneficial as well. This is something that could be added on the end of a therapy day.[8-11]

WHAT IS THE EVIDENCE FOR DURATION OF THERAPY AND MOTOR OUTCOME?

In this day and age of cost-effective care, clinicians sometimes try to get things done as quickly as possible. While there may be short-term benefit, in the long-term that could be quite detrimental.[12] The primary motor cortex is necessary for motor recovery to occur, and if there is a proper activation in therapy this may well improve plasticity within or around the primary cortex.[13] So, we must balance the urge to be cost-effective in the short-term with the long-term outcomes of our patient. We can feel confident that intense repetitive mobility task training is going to benefit our patients. The American Stroke Association/American Heart Association (ASA/AHA) guidelines gave this 1-A evidence. Robotic therapy (RT) and virtual reality technologies, discussed later may be the solution to overcome the limited resources.

WHAT IS OUR APPROACH REGARDING SPECIFIC INTERVENTIONS AND MOTOR DISABILITY?

Let's now look at specific interventions from a physical medicine viewpoint. Ankle-foot orthosis (AFO) can improve gait in patients who may have difficulty during the swing phase of their paretic extremity.[14] The toe can catch, making them more unstable. They also are at risk of developing a plantar flexion contracture at the ankle. An AFO can be very beneficial for this. If the patient is not ambulatory, using a resting ankle splint at night set in neutral is beneficial[15]. A fact too frequently not appreciated by clinicians is that an AFO can improve knee function during ambulation. The hemiparetic leg may be weak, causing the knee to buckle during stance phase. Alternatively, it may be too spastic in extension causing the knee to snap back in genu recurvatum. While a knee orthosis is sometimes used, more effective control can be achieved with an AFO. The collapsing knee can be controlled by putting more plantar flexion into the AFO.[16] This moves the ground reaction force anterior to the knee and adds an extension moment that decreases the tendency to collapse. Conversely, the knee that snaps back into what can be a joint-destroying genu recurvatum can be controlled by putting the AFO into dorsiflexion.[17] This decreases the extension, torch, and increases the flexion moment at the knee, resulting in a more normal gait.

NEWER TECHNOLOGIES AND THEIR EFFECTIVENESS: WHAT IS THE EVIDENCE?

There is no significant evidence to support the use of neuromuscular electrical stimulation (NMES).[18] However, ASA/AHA guidelines do say that NMES or vibration may be a reasonable approach to trying to improve spasticity temporarily. There are few studies in the literature investigating Virtual Reality with electromyographic feedback using visual and auditory signals to improve the patient's muscular activity.[19] A 2007 Cochrane review did not find significant treatment benefits as these studies were small and generally of poor design. In this day and age, virtual reality is becoming a widely used computer technology. This could allow patients to engage in a specific therapeutic task. While the 2011 Cochrane Stroke group concluded there was insufficient evidence to support its use, a recent review showed that virtual reality produces changes in gait parameters despite the fact that it has been poorly standardized in the experimental protocols.[20] There is no question that virtual reality gains in activities are becoming much more widely accessible and there may be significant benefit.

Noninvasive brain stimulation techniques (NIBS) are of two types, Repetitive transcranial magnetic stimulation (rTMS) and transcranial direct current stimulation (tDCS) and these, alter cortical excitability. Transcranial magnetic stimulation induces neuronal depolarization by generating a local magnetic field that creates electrical current to flow through neurons, rTMS is defined as repetition of TMS with high-frequency rTMS causing cortical excitability and low-frequency rTMS suppressing cortical excitability.[21] These techniques in association with RT provide a more precise and quantifiable technology and has shown mixed results in research. Robotic therapy is also useful to calculate the time and dose response with limited resources. Robotic-assisted therapies focus on both upper and lower extremities of the body and allow patients to train independently. Studies using the MIT-MANUS robot developed by the Interactive Motion Technologies Inc., Cambridge, Massachusetts, USA indicate that upper extremity robotic treatment result in improved upper extremity motor recovery compared to traditional rehabilitation therapies. Lokomat (Hocoma Ag, Volketswil, Switzerland) is another robotic-assisted lower extremity device that provide active control at the hip and knee and passive control at the ankle. Studies conducted have shown mixed results and additional trials are needed to confirm the advantages of using robotic-assisted technologies in motor rehabilitation.

EVIDENCE OF PHARMACOLOGICAL MEDICATIONS IN MOTOR RECOVERY FROM STROKE

As a class, SSRIs have varying mechanisms of action that support its role in stroke recovery. These medications promote neuroplasticity. They increase expression of neurotrophins, which induce changes leading to structural adaptation of networks and synapses in response to injury.[22] They promote neurogenesis in the subependymal region and subgranular area of the hippocampal dentate gyrus.[23] In the subacute to late stage after an ischemic stroke, at the cellular level, inflammation contributes to cellular injury. Serotonin reuptake inhibitors inhibit neutrophil granulocytes and microglia.[24] In rat models for ischemic stroke, this results in a reduction of the infarct size. Following administration of SSRIs, increased levels of vascular endothelial growth factor, a protective agent, are noted.[22] Other experiments have shown an upregulation of β-1 adrenergic system within the caudate, putamen, and frontal lobes following administration of SSRIs.[22] Use of functional MRI methods showed that stroke patients have increased excitation of the motor cortex after administration of fluoxetine.[25]

Fluoxetine for motor recovery after acute ischemic stroke (FLAME) trial was a double blind placebo controlled trial conducted in France.[26] A total of 118 patients with ischemic stroke and moderate to severe motor deficit (Fugl-Meyer motor scale score of 55 or less) were randomly assigned to fluoxetine 20 mg once a day versus placebo in combination with physical therapy. The medication was started within 5–10 days after stroke onset and continued for 90 days.[26] The improvement in Fugl-Meyer motor scale scores was significantly higher in the fluoxetine group compared with placebo (34.0 versus 24.3, p = 0.003).[26] The proposed mechanism of benefit was modulation of spontaneous brain plasticity.[26] This trial confirmed the relatively consistent benefit from fluoxetine noted in several prior, smaller studies.

Poststroke depression occurs in about one-third of ischemic stroke patients. One explanation could be that SSRIs improve participation in rehabilitation by improving mood and motivation among patients. In the FLAME trial, after adjustment for clinical depression diagnosed before day 90, the change in Fugl-Meyer motor scale was still significantly better among the fluoxetine group compared with placebo.[26] Therefore, the benefit from SSRIs seems to be beyond the improvement of clinical depression.

Dopamine is an important neurotransmitter that regulates movement, reward, learning, and neuroplasticity. Dopamine is essential for learning of motor skills by its influence on cortical plasticity. Therefore, L-dopa has been tested in motor recovery from stroke. In a prospective randomized, placebo-controlled, double blind study, 53 patients with stroke were administered L-dopa 100 mg daily versus placebo in combination with physical therapy for 3 weeks.[27] Motor recovery, measured by the Rivermead motor assessment (RMA) was significantly better in the L-dopa group ($p < 0.004$). This benefit was maintained at 3 weeks after L-dopa was discontinued in the trial ($p = 0.02$).[27] Larger studies using L-dopa are needed to routinely recommend it among patients with stroke.

Amphetamines have been tried in stroke recovery; however, the data regarding their benefit is inconsistent. In a single, small study of ten hemiplegic patients with an ischemic stroke; 10 mg of D-amphetamine versus placebo was administered with physical therapy for ten doses every 4th day. There was a significant benefit in the amphetamine group in the Fugl-Meyer motor score. The benefit was noted at 1 week and at the 12 month follow-up visit ($p = 0.047$).[28] This benefit was not borne out in several subsequent studies. In one trial, 24 stroke patients were randomized to receive 10 mg of D-amphetamine or placebo every 4th day, combined with physical therapy within 60 minutes after drug intake. The trial was conducted within 6 weeks after the stroke and continued for 36 days (total 100 mg D-amphetamine).[29] The active drug group did not show any significant differences in improvement of activities of daily living (Barthel index) compared with placebo.[29]

Another small trial failed to show benefit of amphetamines in promoting motor performance during training sessions, skill acquisition with training tasks, and motor recovery among stroke patients with mild arm weakness.[30] In a relatively large randomized double blind, placebo controlled trial in 71 stroke patients with severe motor deficits; 10 mg of amphetamine was coupled with physical therapy twice a week for 5 weeks in the early post stroke period. Compared with placebo, however showed no significant differences in recovery.[31] In another placebo controlled trial, patients were randomized to either 20 mg of D-amphetamine, 100 mg of L-dopa or a combination of 10 mg of D-amphetamine with 50 mg of L-dopa, combined with physical therapy. The active drug arms did not show any benefit over physical therapy alone in recovery of motor function or activities of daily living.[32] Based on these negative studies, the routine use of amphetamines to promote motor recovery cannot be recommended.

WHAT IS SPASTICITY? CAN WE TREAT THIS CONDITION?

Spasticity, which is classically defined as velocity-dependent resistance to stretch, occurs in the upper motor neuron syndrome seen in stroke. Spasticity can increase the cost of care, although it may be secondary to its reflexion of the stroke severity.[33,34] As stated above, the use of AFOs can help spasticity in the lower extremity from turning into contractures. However, the use of resting hand splints has not been shown to be effective for reducing wrist and finger spasticity. The use of such splints at best, is controversial.[35] Stretching can be important, particularly when it is done in a slow and controlled manner. This has been well demonstrated in the shoulder. Positioning of the hemiplegic shoulder in maximal external rotation while the patient is either sitting or in bed for 30 minutes daily can be helpful.[4] Baclofen and the traditional muscle relaxants have been used in reducing the muscle tone and improving spasticity. More literature is available and is beyond the scope of this review.

MOBILITY AND STROKE

Mobility is obviously an important part of recovery from stroke. These include activities such as going from lying in bed to sitting at the side of the bed to standing from sitting to transferring, such as from wheelchair to bed or bed to chair, turning, ambulation, and even advanced techniques, such as stair climbing. With impairments of mobility, there is increased risk of fall. As previously stated, intensity of treatment is very important. Use of AFO may be very helpful. However, there is no benefit from more advanced or complex techniques, such as treadmill or robotic-based interventions compared with traditional treatment approaches. They are still under evaluation.[36] The ongoing studies are showing that there may be benefit in these techniques if they could increase the amount of the desired pattern.[37]

HOW CAN WE APPROACH DECONDITIONING AND FITNESS IN STROKE PATIENTS?

While we focus primarily on the stroke's impact on its vocal areas, it is important to keep an eye on the whole person. There is no question that people with stroke tend to have impaired fitness levels. For example, they may have a peak VO_2 max of only 8–20 mL of oxygen per kg/minute which is only 53% of age and sex matched controls.[38] Now to be able to participate in independent living, it is often thought that a person needs at least 15–18 mL of oxygen per kg/minute. Therefore, the poor level of fitness after a stroke can cause significant health and functional quality problems.[39] It is so important to keep people active as activity level is a predictor of life satisfaction.[40] Therefore, working on aerobic activity after strokes will have significant health benefits both in the physical and psychosocial domains. We often hear complaints of our stroke patients about fatigue and depression, emotional wellbeing.[41,42] Being in better shape may even help improvement in walking and upper extremity muscle strength.[43]

DOES RECREATION PLAY A ROLE?

Recreation has often been neglected in stroke rehab. There are obviously many things that are focused on. However, a key thing to remember in stroke rehab is that it is crucial to get the patient invested in his or her therapy. A person who has no place to go is not going to be interested in gait training. A person who has no reason to get dressed is not going to be interested in activities of daily living. If we can find things that are important and meaningful for the person, recreation may be one of these avenues. It will help in improving overall outcomes.[44]

CONCLUSION

To conclude, a key point when looking at physical medicine modalities and rehabilitation after stroke is that it must be tailored according to the individual. We have to see how the person responds. This can help us in developing proper repetition, aggressive task difficulty, and functional practice of important activities.[45] As stated earlier, standard prescription of exercise, such as the mode, frequency, duration, and intensity require careful application so it is safe intervention that accommodates the individual with his or her functional limitations, motivation, comorbidities, and very importantly individual goals. While we are looking at the entire stroke population, we must remember that there are individuals who may vary within this population and just as in any type of deficit, we have to monitor how the patient is doing and adjust it appropriately to maximize the level of improvement. Just as care is taken with prescribing a particular medicine, precision and care must be taken while prescribing a rehabilitation modality.

REFERENCES

1. Benjamin EJ, Virani SS, Callaway CW, et al. Heart disease and stroke statistics-2018 update: A report from the American Heart Association. Circulation. 2018;137:e67-492.
2. Cramer SC. Repairing the human brain after stroke. II. Restorative therapies. Ann Neurol. 2008;63:549-60.
3. DeJong G, Horn SD, Conroy B, et al. Opening the black box of post-stroke rehabilitation: stroke rehabilitation patients, processes, and outcomes. Arch Phys Med Rehabil. 2005;86:S1-7.
4. Winstein CJ, Stein J, Arena R, et al. Guidelines for adult stroke rehabilitation and recovery: A guideline for healthcare professionals from the American Heart Association/American Stroke Association. Stroke. 2016;47:e98-169.
5. Hornby TG, Holleran CL, Hennessy PW, et al. Variable intensive early walking poststroke (VIEWS): A randomized controlled trial. Neurorehabil Neural Repair. 2016;30:440-50.
6. Moore JL, Roth EJ, Killian C, et al. Locomotor training improves daily stepping activity and gait efficiency in individuals poststroke who have reached a "plateau" in recovery. Stroke. 2010;41:129-35.
7. Lang CE, Macdonald JR, Reisman DS, et al. Observation of amounts of movement practice provided during stroke rehabilitation. Arch Phys Med Rehabil. 2009;90:1692-8.
8. Dromerick AW, Lang CE, Birkenmeier RL, et al. Very early constraint-induced movement during stroke rehabilitation (VECTORS): A single-center RCT. Neurology 2009;73:195-201.
9. Boake C, Noser EA, Ro T, et al. Constraint-induced movement therapy during early stroke rehabilitation. Neurorehabil Neural Repair. 2007;21:14-24.
10. Page SJ, Levine P, Leonard A, et al. Modified constraint-induced therapy in chronic stroke: Results of a single-blinded randomized controlled trial. Phys Ther. 2008;88:333-40.
11. Page SJ, Levine P, Leonard AC. Modified constraint-induced therapy in acute stroke: a randomized controlled pilot study. Neurorehabil Neural Repair. 2005;19:27-32.
12. Roby-Brami A, Feydy A, Combeaud M, et al. Motor compensation and recovery for reaching in stroke patients. Acta Neurol Scand. 2003;107:369-81.
13. Liepert J, Bauder H, Wolfgang HR, et al. Treatment-induced cortical reorganization after stroke in humans. Stroke. 2000;31:1210-6.
14. Nonnekes J, Benda N, van Duijnhoven H, et al. Management of gait impairments in chronic unilateral upper motor neuron lesions: A review. JAMA Neurol. 2018;75:751-8.
15. Robinson W, Smith R, Aung O, Ada L. No difference between wearing a night splint and standing on a tilt table in preventing ankle contracture early after stroke: A randomised trial. Aust J Physiother. 2008;54:33-8.
16. DeLisa J. Rehabilitation medicine: Principles and practice. Philadelphia: Lippincott, 1998.
17. Ohsawa S, Ikeda S, Tanaka S, et al. A new model of plastic ankle foot orthosis (FAFO (II)) against spastic foot and genu recurvatum. Prosthet Orthot Int. 1992;16:104-8.
18. Sabut SK, Sikdar C, Kumar R, et al. Functional electrical stimulation of dorsiflexor muscle: Effects on dorsiflexor strength, plantarflexor spasticity, and motor recovery in stroke patients. Neuro Rehabilitation. 2011;29:393-400.
19. Saposnik G, Teasell R, Mamdani M, et al. Effectiveness of virtual reality using Wii gaming technology in stroke rehabilitation: A pilot randomized clinical trial and proof of principle. Stroke. 2010;41:1477-84.
20. Moreira MC, de Amorim Lima AM, Ferraz KM, et al. Use of virtual reality in gait recovery among post

stroke patients--a systematic literature review. Disabil Rehabil Assist Technol. 2013;8:357-62.
21. Simonetta-Moreau M. Non-invasive brain stimulation (NIBS) and motor recovery after stroke. Ann Phys Rehabil Med. 2014;57:530-42.
22. Siepmann T, Penzlin AI, Kepplinger J, et al. Selective serotonin reuptake inhibitors to improve outcome in acute ischemic stroke: Possible mechanisms and clinical evidence. Brain Behav. 2015;5:e00373.
23. Li WL, Cai HH, Wang B, et al. Chronic fluoxetine treatment improves ischemia-induced spatial cognitive deficits through increasing hippocampal neurogenesis after stroke. J Neurosci Res. 2009;87:112-22.
24. Lim CM, Kim SW, Park JY, Kim C, Yoon SH, Lee JK. Fluoxetine affords robust neuroprotection in the postischemic brain via its anti-inflammatory effect. J Neurosci Res 2009;87:1037-45.
25. Dam M, Tonin P, De Boni A, et al. Effects of fluoxetine and maprotiline on functional recovery in poststroke hemiplegic patients undergoing rehabilitation therapy. Stroke 1996;27:1211-4.
26. Chollet F, Tardy J, Albucher JF, et al. Fluoxetine for motor recovery after acute ischaemic stroke (FLAME): A randomised placebo-controlled trial. Lancet Neurol;10:123-30.
27. Scheidtmann K, Fries W, Muller F, Koenig E. Effect of levodopa in combination with physiotherapy on functional motor recovery after stroke: A prospective, randomised, double-blind study. Lancet. 2001;358:787-90.
28. Walker-Batson D, Smith P, Curtis S, et al. Amphetamine paired with physical therapy accelerates motor recovery after stroke. Further evidence. Stroke 1995;26:2254-9.
29. Treig T, Werner C, Sachse M, et al. No benefit from D-amphetamine when added to physiotherapy after stroke: A randomized, placebo-controlled study. Clin Rehabil. 2003;17:590-9.
30. Platz T, Kim IH, Engel U, et al. Amphetamine fails to facilitate motor performance and to enhance motor recovery among stroke patients with mild arm paresis: Interim analysis and termination of a double blind, randomised, placebo-controlled trial. Restor Neurol Neurosci. 2005;23:271-80.
31. Gladstone DJ, Danells CJ, Armesto A, et al. Physiotherapy coupled with dextroamphetamine for rehabilitation after hemiparetic stroke: A randomized, double-blind, placebo-controlled trial. Stroke. 2006;37:179-85.
32. Sonde L, Lokk J. Effects of amphetamine and/or L-dopa and physiotherapy after stroke - a blinded randomized study. Acta Neurol Scand. 2007;115:55-9.
33. Lundstrom E, Smits A, Borg J, et al. Four-fold increase in direct costs of stroke survivors with spasticity compared with stroke survivors without spasticity: The first year after the event. Stroke. 2010;41:319-24.
34. Urban PP, Wolf T, Uebele M, et al. Occurence and clinical predictors of spasticity after ischemic stroke. Stroke. 2010;41:2016-20.
35. Basaran A, Emre U, Karadavut KI, et al. Hand splinting for poststroke spasticity: a randomized controlled trial. Top Stroke Rehabil. 2012;19:329-37.
36. Dobkin BH, Duncan PW. Should body weight-supported treadmill training and robotic-assistive steppers for locomotor training trot back to the starting gate? Neurorehabil Neural Repair. 2012;26:308-17.
37. Hornby TG, Moore JL, Lovell L, et al. Influence of skill and exercise training parameters on locomotor recovery during stroke rehabilitation. Curr Opin Neurol. 2016;29:677-83.
38. Smith AC, Saunders DH, Mead G. Cardiorespiratory fitness after stroke: A systematic review. Int J Stroke. 2012;7:499-510.
39. Shephard RJ. Maximal oxygen intake and independence in old age. Br J Sports Med. 2009;43:342-6.
40. Hartman-Maeir A, Soroker N, Ring H, et al. Activities, participation and satisfaction one-year post stroke. Disabil Rehabil. 2007;29:559-66.
41. Zedlitz AM, Rietveld TC, Geurts AC, et al. Cognitive and graded activity training can alleviate persistent fatigue after stroke: A randomized, controlled trial. Stroke. 2012;43:1046-51.
42. Stuart M, Benvenuti F, Macko R, et al. Community-based adaptive physical activity program for chronic stroke: feasibility, safety, and efficacy of the Empoli model. Neurorehabil Neural Repair. 2009;23:726-34.
43. Harris JE, Eng JJ. Strength training improves upper-limb function in individuals with stroke: A meta-analysis. Stroke. 2010;41:136-40.
44. Richter KJ, Sherrill, C, McCann, BC, et al. Physical Medicine and Rehabilitation Principles and Practice. Recreation and Sport for People with Disabilities. Philadelphia: Lippincott-Williams & Wilkins, 2005.
45. Management of Stroke Rehabilitation Working Group. VA/DOD Clinical practice guideline for the management of stroke rehabilitation. J Rehabil Res Dev. 2010;47:1-43.

CHAPTER 12

Current Role of Statins in Cerebrovascular Diseases

Meenakshisundaram U, Sreenivas UM

INTRODUCTION

Statins have been used as a vital part of stroke management strategies for a long while. Statins were primarily developed as a lipid-lowering drug (LLD) to combat atherosclerosis, which is one of the most common mechanisms of stroke. However, recent evidence is emerging that statins have a role in stroke that go beyond simple lipid lowering and its attendant benefits.

Clinical trials have shown a protective effect of statins in stroke, when started either before or immediately after the cerebral artery occlusion. This has shown a significant reduction in infarct volume and improved outcomes in studies involving animals. In this chapter, we will look into the varied benefits of statins in cerebrovascular disease.

MECHANISM OF ACTION

Inhibition of Cholesterol Synthesis

The primary action of statins is to decrease generation of serum low-density lipoprotein (LDL). This in turn leads to decreased rates of atherosclerosis and vessel occlusion. This effect is mediated by the inhibition of 3-hydroxy-3-methylglutaryl-coenzyme A (HMG-CoA) reductase enzyme, which is the rate limiting enzyme in cholesterol synthesis.

This hepatic cholesterol synthesis is responsible for almost two-thirds of serum cholesterol.[1]

The decrease in LDL cholesterol may in turn lead to an upregulation of LDL-receptors, with resultant increase in LDL clearance from the blood.[1] Lower levels of LDL contribute to a delay in atherosclerotic plaque growth, leading to lower risk of cerebrovascular and cardiovascular events.[2]

Inhibition of Isoprenoid Synthesis

The action on HMG-CoA reductase also results in decreased production of other cholesterol-dependent intermediate metabolites, important among which are isoprenoids.

The isoprenoids are important in cellular signaling for cell proliferation, differentiation and migration. They are important moieties in the post-translational modification of proteins such as G-proteins and GTP-binding molecules. Ras, Rho, Rap, and Rab GTPases are dependent on modification of farnesyl diphosphate and geranylgeranyl pyrophosphate.[2] Statins inhibit this process by inhibiting farnesylation and geranylgeranylation through isoprenylation. This prevents activation of the signaling molecules.[1] This in turn leads to increased endothelial nitric oxide synthase (eNOS) activity and decreased NADPH (nicotinamide adenine dinucleotide phosphate) oxidase and superoxide activation, decreasing inactivation of NO. This enhances NO activity leads to improvement in cardiovascular function, through decreased platelet activation and suppression of inflammatory cascade.[1] This benefit might even predate the reduction of cholesterol levels in the blood.[2]

Stabilization of Plaque

The statins have an action on the atherosclerosis by stabilizing the plaque and activating fibrinolysis. The suppression of inflammatory cascade and immunomodulation have an important role in this action. This suppression may be objectively demonstrated by the lowering of C-reactive protein (CRP) levels in patients treated with statins.[1]

Anti-inflammatory Effects

Reactive oxygen species (ROS) have been shown to cause neuronal tissue damage. This is shown to be increased by risk factors such as diabetes mellitus, smoking, metabolic syndrome, hypercholesterolemia, and hypertension. The ROS accelerate atherosclerosis causing progressive cerebrovascular damage. The statins have an indirect inhibitory action on the production of ROS via inhibiting NADPHase and stimulating NO synthesis.[2]

Atorvastatin has been shown to upregulate catalase expression without affecting superoxide dismutase (SOD) and glutathione peroxidase (GPx) expression. This effect is seen in endothelial cells in humans.[3] Simvastatin has been shown to stimulate heme oxygenase, which is an effective antioxidant, in vascular smooth muscle cells. These actions aid in scavenging of free radicals and thus help to prevent acceleration of atherosclerosis.

The animal models have also demonstrated an effect of statins on the stiffness of vessel walls by acting on the Cu/ZnSOD and increasing its activity and consequently reducing superoxide production.[2]

Nicotinamide adenine dinucleotide phosphate oxidase is a prominent source of free radicals. The inhibition of this enzyme by statins has been shown through multiple studies. Statins specifically inhibit and down-regulate the Nox1 and Nox2 isoforms, although some studies have also suggested an action on Nox4 isoforms. The effect is mediated through down regulation of the mRNA for the specific isoforms. This effect is pronounced in the cells of the vascular tissue.[3] The inhibition of NADPH oxidase in THP-1 monocytes is of particular interest, given the role of these cells in the pathogenesis and growth of atherosclerotic plaques.[4]

Modulation of Nitric Oxide Synthesis

The eNOS is an integral part of the protective mechanism for vascular endothelium. It is paradoxically up-regulated by oxidative stress. Raised NO is shown to improve endothelial function. Statins increase activity of eNOS in multiple ways. Phosphorylation of the eNOS at Ser633 and Ser1177 have been shown to increase acetylcholine-induced vasodilation. Statins are also shown to increase tetrahydrobiopterin (BH4) biosynthesis by activating GTP cyclohydrolase I.[4,5] The BH4 is a vital cofactor in the generation of NO. Stability of NO is also supposed to be increased by statins via action on their mRNA. Thus statins have a combined effect of increased NO activity.[5]

Inducible NOS (iNOS) have the opposite effect to eNOS and contribute to neuronal degeneration and oxidise structure neuronal proteins. This enzyme is inducible by ischemia. Statins have been shown to inhibit the cytokine mediated up-regulation of iNOS following stroke. This helps to restrict the ischemic damage to neuronal tissue.

Stabilization of Blood–Brain Barrier

Matrix metalloproteinases (MMPs) are known to be a critical enzyme in the pathogenesis of atherosclerotic plaques. They are also considered to be the part of the pathogenesis of multiple neurological disorders such as multiple sclerosis, stroke, and spinal cord injury. The enzyme, MMP-9, is released from nervous tissue following ischemic insult and can lead to breakdown of the blood–brain barrier (BBB). This leads to impaired perfusion of the normal tissue and can lead to propagation of the insult. This has a role in stroke thrombolysis[6,7] as well since the disruption of the BBB can lead to higher chances of hemorrhagic transformation and clinical deterioration. Statins have been shown to inhibit this enzyme. Animal studies have shown a benefit of using recombinant tissue plasminogen activator along with statins to decrease the risk of hemorrhagic transformation and prolonging the window period for thrombolysis beyond 3 hours.[5]

Angiogenesis

Atorvastatin is *in vivo* metabolized to hydroxy products. These products have been shown in mice to promote angiogenesis and brain plasticity following stroke, through induction of vascular endothelial growth factor and brain-derived neurotrophic factor. This is another possible mechanism contributing to the neuroprotective effect of statins.[3]

Statins also a protective antithrombotic effect on platelets by decreasing the production of thromboxane A2 in erythrocyte and platelet membranes. This leads to a decreased thrombogenic state.[1] Statins have also been found to increase thrombomodulin expression, which inhibits thrombosis.

Although we have discussed many of the proposed and proven mechanisms of action of statins, we have not been able to fully and comprehensively understand the pleiotropic effects of statin on neurological tissue and this subject warrants further research.

PHARMACOKINETICS

Statins can be classified based on their manufacture as naturally derived (type 1) and synthetic (type 2). The naturally derived statins are usually extracted from certain fermented fungi. These two types vary considerably in their structures and physical properties. Type 2 are typically lipophilic and can cross the BBB. This leads to higher neuroprotective effects of type 2 statins compared to type 1.[6] Type 2 includes atorvastatin, rosuvastatin and fluvastatin. In addition simvastatin of type 1 statins are also lipophilic and share many of the properties and actions of type 2 statins. Despite these differences, all types of statins act primarily on a single target molecule, HMG-CoA reductase.

CLINICAL APPLICATIONS

Statins have been used in neurology primarily for the management of stroke. The rationale for the use of statins has been proven by a beneficial outcomes of multiple trials.

Ischemic Stroke

Ischemic stroke is the most common type of cerebrovascular disease. It can be thrombotic or embolic and have high morbidity and mortality rates. Risk factor modification is the primary target of stroke prevention and management. Among the known and proven risk factors, control of elevated blood cholesterol is the second most efficacious intervention, superseded only by blood pressure control.[8] There are no studies showing conclusive evidence of the causative effect of high cholesterol in stroke. However, the Multiple Risk Factor Intervention Trial has shown a correlation between higher cholesterol levels and higher mortality and morbidity of ischemic strokes. The Stroke Prevention by Aggressive Reduction of Cholesterol Levels (SPARCLE) is the first study to prospectively prove the beneficial effects of atorvastatin in stroke. It showed a reduction in stroke of 12–16%.[8] Multiple studies including the WOS-COPS, CARE and LIPID studies have shown stroke prevention from statins to be ranging from 10–30%.[9] However a meta-analysis of studies on statins in acute ischemic stroke could not demonstrate any benefit in RCTs. However, this could be confounded by the small sample sizes in the randomized controlled trials (RCTs). Further studies have shown a correlation between statin use following stroke and better clinical outcomes, depending on the severity of the stroke. This effect is especially pronounced if statin is started after the first ever ischemic stroke.

The PROSPER (Patient-Centered Research into Outcomes Stroke Patients Prefer and Effectiveness Research) trial looked into the real world effectiveness of use of statins for secondary prevention of ischemic stroke. Two years follow-up with statins showed a significant reduction in major cardiac adverse events, all-cause mortality and all cause readmission. However, risk of recurrence of ischemic stroke or hemorrhagic stroke did not change with use of statins. There was no difference in the outcomes between high intensity and moderate intensity statin therapy groups of the trial. This shows that the beneficial effects of statins are not dose dependent.[8]

Nonminor strokes derive maximum benefit from statin use, with a proven reduction in mortality and morbidity rates. Secondary prevention with statins is recommended after the first ischemic stroke or transient ischemic event. Statin use showed a marked reduction in the number of transient ischemic attacks (TIAs). Pretreatment with statins has also shown a reduction in stroke severity with a reduction in infarct size of almost 30%.[9] Statins are effective in both thrombotic and embolic strokes. In thrombotic strokes, the atherosclerosis of the affected vessel will be stabilized and suppressed by statins leading to decreased thrombotic rates. In embolus, the source of emboli is usually a larger vessel upstream from an atherosclerotic plaque. The pleomorphic effects of the statins on these plaques thus prevents artery-to-artery embolism. The inhibitory effects on MMP-9 is also protective following intravenous thrombolysis and in the initial period following a stroke by preventing hemorrhagic transformation and extension of the infarct.[9]

Stabilization of plaque is the most obvious mechanism of action. Statins affect two of the major components of plaque formation-cholesterol deposition and macrophage foam cell formation, via inhibition of MMPs. Decreased platelet activity is another proposed action, with reduced platelet aggregation and thromboxane production. A reduction in platelet membrane cholesterol levels is cited as the possible reason for these effects.

A meta-analysis of multiple trials of statin usage in ischemic stroke by Arboix et al. in 2016 concurred with the benefits described above. However, it did not show any benefit on functional outcomes at 1-year after stroke.[9] It also reinforced the benefits of pretreatment with statins before stroke and simultaneous usage of statins in intravenous thrombolysis. However this also suggested a potentially higher incidence of stroke and stroke related mortality following statin usage, in patients who are post renal transplant or on regular hemodialysis. This meta-analysis also cautioned against the use of statins in strokes of unusual cause.[9]

Apart from these effects, a study by Guo J et al. published in 2015 showed that statin use following an ischemic stroke helped to decrease the incidence of early poststroke seizures. It also showed a possible benefit in reducing the progression of poststroke seizures into chronic epilepsy. These results had a level of evidence of Class III.[10]

Statins may be used as high intensity, moderate intensity or low intensity. This differentiation is as follows:

- *High intensity*: Atorvastatin 80 mg, rosuvastatin 20 mg
- *Moderate intensity*: Atorvastatin 40 mg, rosuvastatin 10 mg, and simvastatin 40 mg
- *Low intensity*: Atorvastatin 20 mg, rosuvastatin 5 mg, and pitavastatin 4 mg.

The recent 2018 American Heart Association (AHA) guidelines for acute stroke recommend the following:[11]

- If a patient is already on statins at the time of onset of ischemic stroke, continue the statins—Class IIa
- High-intensity statin therapy should be initiated or continued in patients ≤75 years of age who have clinical ASCVD (Atherosclerotic Cardiovascular Disease), unless contraindicated—Class I. If a patient with clinical ASCVD has contraindications for high-intensity statins or has a high risk for statin related adverse effects, moderate intensity statins are to be used if tolerated—Class I
- If the patient with clinical ASCVD is aged >75 years, it is reasonable to evaluate the risk-reduction benefits, adverse effects, and drug-drug interactions when initiating a high-intensity or moderate-intensity statin. If the patients is already tolerating statin, it is reasonable to continue the same—Class IIb

- Patients with ischemic stroke and other comorbid ASCVD should be managed with lifestyle modification, dietary recommendations and medications—Class I
- In patients with acute ischemic stroke, who qualify for statin use, in-hospital initiation of statins is reasonable—Class IIa.

The 2016 ESC/EAS guidelines for management of dyslipidemias recommends that intensive statin therapy be initiated in all patients with a history of noncardioembolic ischemic stroke or TIA.

The 2013 ACC/AHA guidelines on treatment of blood cholesterol suggests that a single fixed dose of statins be used. There was no target for reduction of LDL cholesterol.

In contrast, the Canadian Cardiovascular Society recommends a target LDL-C level <2.0 mmol/L or a >50% reduction in LDL-C.[11]

Future direction for statin therapy include a possible benefit of adding other LLDs to statins such as ezetimbe and PCSK9 inhibitors. Further studies for the same are warranted.

Hemorrhagic Stroke

Hemorrhagic strokes are less common compared to their ischemic counterparts. They can be parenchymal or subarachnoid hemorrhages (SAHs). The role of statins in hemorrhagic stroke is controversial. Studies such as SPARCL have reported an increased risk of hemorrhagic stroke associated with low cholesterol values, especially LDL. Total cholesterol is found to have an inverse relationship with the risk of hemorrhage and microbleeds.[12] This correlation is much more robust in women. Higher levels of LDL and higher non-high-density lipoprotein (HDL) to HDL ratio are found to be associated with lower risk of hemorrhagic stroke. This would rule out any role for statins, seeing as their primary role seems to be detrimental in this condition. However, higher triglyceride levels are also associated with an increased risk of hemorrhage. A study by Ma et al. published in 2016 has shown no concrete evidence of increase in hemorrhage associated with use of statins.[12] However in elderly patients with poorly controlled hypertension, the use of statins at high doses is associated with a significantly higher risk of intracerebral hemorrhage. Recent studies have shown an encouraging effect and improved outcomes of statins in hemorrhagic stroke. Pretreatment with statins has been found useful even in this type of stroke. Furthermore, statins also have an antivasospasm effect and can delay ischemic insult in patients with SAH. Serum markers of brain injury are consequently much lower following statin use.[9]

ADVERSE EFFECTS

Despite the high incidence of beneficial effects of statins, adverse effects are not uncommon and a clinician requires knowledge of these effects to be able to recognize them. This is particularly common when the statins are used alongside another class of LLDs.

Cholesterol synthesis inhibition has led to induction of apoptosis of cells in neuronal and glial culture tissues. This effect is attributed to decreased isoprenylation, by inhibition of the isoprenoid pathway. This process is important for the activation of molecules involved in regulation of cell proliferation.[9]

Multiple systemic side effects are also noted. The chief among them are the presence of myopathy and liver toxicity. The severity of these effects is usually minimal and benign. However they can be severe leading to rhabdomyolysis and consequent renal failure. This effect is more common when statins are combined with other LLDs.[9] The singular characteristic of this myopathy is its resolution on cessation of the drug.

CONCLUSION

Statins are the second most important drug in stroke management after the time window has elapsed, superseded only by aspirin. It is primarily a LLD that, through the years, has been demonstrated to have multiple "pleiotropic" effects, which have been shown to be neuroprotective independent of the cholesterol levels. Statins are now standardly used in all ischemic strokes, where it has a number of effects to prevent tissue damage and aid recovery. The optimum dosage of statins is one which confers maximal benefit without adverse effects. Further studies are needed to elicit the exact mechanism of action of statins causing the pleiomorphic effects and also to determine the optimal doses of the various statins. Statin is a drug of the past, present, and the future.

REFERENCES

1. Malfitano A, Marasco G, Proto M, et al. Statins in neurological disorders: An overview and update. Pharmacological Research. 2014;88:74-83.
2. Zhao J, Zhang X, Dong L, et al. The many roles of statins in ischemic stroke. Current Neuropharmacology. 2015;12(6):564-74.
3. Hong K, Lee J. Statins in acute ischemic stroke: A systematic review. J Stroke. 2015;17(3):282-301.
4. Miida T, Hirayama S, Nakamura Y. Cholesterol-independent effects of statins and new therapeutic targets: Ischemic stroke and dementia. J Atheroscler Thromb. 2004;11(5):253-64.
5. Castilla-Guerra L, del Carmen Fernandez-Moreno M, Angel Colmenero-Camacho M. Statins in stroke prevention: Present and future. Current pharmaceutical design. 2016;22(30):4638-44.
6. Ling Q, Tejada-Simon M. Statins and the brain: New perspective for old drugs. Prog Neuro-Psychopharmacol Biol Psychiatry. 2016;66:80-6.
7. Schmeer C, Kretz A, Isenmann S. Statin-mediated protective effects in the central nervous system: General mechanisms and putative role of stress proteins. Restor Neurol Neurosci. 2006;24(2):79-95.
8. O'Brien E, Greiner M, Xian Y, et al. Clinical effectiveness of statin therapy after ischemic stroke: Primary Results From the Statin Therapeutic Area of the Patient-Centered Research Into Outcomes Stroke Patients Prefer and Effectiveness Research (PROSPER) study clinical perspective. Circulation. 2015;132(15):1404-13.
9. Arboix A, Rosselló-Vicens G, Sánchez M. Statin therapy for stroke prevention: Current status and controversies. International Journal of Cardiology and Lipidology Research. 2016;3(1):1-5.
10. Guo J, Guo J, Li J, et al. Statin treatment reduces the risk of poststroke seizures. Neurology. 2015;85(8):701-7.
11. Powers W, Rabinstein A, Ackerson T, et al. 2018 Guidelines for the early management of patients with acute ischemic stroke: A Guideline for healthcare professionals from the American Heart Association/American Stroke Association. Stroke. 2018;49(3):e46-99.
12. Ma Y, Li Z, Chen L, et al. Blood lipid levels, statin therapy and the risk of intracerebral hemorrhage. Lipids Health Dis. 2016;15:43.

INDEX

Page numbers followed by *b* refer to box, *f* refer to figure, *fc* refer to flowchart, and *t* refer to table.

A

Acetaminophen 88
Acetylcholine 7
Acquired epileptic aphasia 23
Actinomyces israelii 36
Actinomycosis 36
Adrenergic antagonists 8
Agnosia training 69
Alexia 70
Alfuzosin 8
Alveolaris 42
Alzheimer's disease 58
Amantadine 95
Amikacin 41
Amino acids 49
Amphotericin
   B 41
     deoxycholate 46
     lipid complex 44, 46
     lipid formulation of 46
Amyloidosis 13
Ankle-foot orthosis 117
Anterolisthesis, grade 2 83f
Antibiotic 34, 41
   therapy, long-term 39
Anticholinergics 95
Antidromic sensory recording 14
Antiepileptic medications 28
   role of 28
Antifungal therapy 49
Anti-inflammatory effects 124
Antimuscarinic drugs 7, 7t
Antineutophilic cytoplasmic
     antibody 51
   associated diseases 51
Antiparkinsonian medications 74
Anti-siphon devices 63
Anxiety 28
Apathy 95
Apophysomyces 45
Apparent disc herniation 83f
Apraxia
   interventions for functional
     limitations to 69
   training 68
Arachnoid cyst 83f
Artery thrombosis, median 13
Aspergillosis 48
Aspergillus fumigatus 48
Astereognosis 70
Astrocytoma 82f
Atherosclerotic plaques 124
Atorvastatin 124, 125
Atrial fibrillation 108
Attention deficits 67, 68
Audiovestibular damage 50
Auricular chondritis, bilateral 50
Autoimmune thyroid disease 112
Autoimmune thyroiditis 112
Automatic brain systems 67
Autonomic nervous system 74
Azathioprine 50, 51
Azithromycin 39, 41
Azoles
   like fluconazole 41
   like voriconazole 49

B

Babinski sign 91
Back pain, without 85fc
Baclofen 8
Bacterial infections 33
Balamuthia mandrillaris 41
Bartonella henselae 39
Basedow's paraparesis 109
Behavioral techniques 5
Behçet's disease 51
Benzodiazepines 8
Birbeck granules 54
Bladder
   dysfunction 2f
   expression 6
   innervation, anatomy of 1, 1f
   neck dyssynergia 3
   reflex, cortical regulation of 3
   sphincter procedure 9
Blake's pouch cyst 58
Blood
   pressure 105t
     increasing 95
Blood-brain barrier 124
   stabilization of 124
Body bradykinesia 104
Botulinum toxin 9
Brachial plexopathy 13, 16
Bradykinesia 73, 75, 91, 98
Bragard's sign 85
Brain
   stimulation techniques 70
   tumor cortical trauma 3
Broca's area 70
Brucellosis 34
Buddha's hand appearance 40, 40f

C

Candidiasis 47
Carbimazole 109
Cardiopulmonary impairment 97
Carpal tunnel 12
   cross sectional anatomy of 12f
   lipoma 13
   surface anatomy of 12f
   surgical decompression of 18f
   syndrome 12, 13, 13b, 14t, 16, 16b, 17, 111
   grading severity of 14t
Caspofungin 49
Cat scratch disease 39
Cauda equina syndrome 1, 81f
Ceftriaxone 34
Cell proliferation, regulation of 127
Central disc herniation 81f
Central nervous system 31, 33, 34, 36, 37, 47, 48, 51

toxoplasmosis 42
Centro temporal
  electrodes 24f
  spikes 23, 24f
Cerebellar atrophy 54
Cerebral
  abscesses 37, 47
  artery, middle 35, 42
  paragonimasis 40
  recovery after stroke 65fc
  schistosomiasis 40
  syphilitic gumma 36
Cerebrospinal fluid 34, 39, 41, 42f, 44, 57
  block, complete 87f
  flow 61
  outflow studies 62
Cerebrovascular accidents 108
Cerebrovascular diseases, current role of statins in 123
Cervical radiculopathy 13
Childhood epilepsy, benign 23
Chlorambucil 51
Cholesterol
  levels, aggressive reduction of 125
  synthesis 127
    enzyme in 123
    inhibition of 123
Cholestyramine 110
Cholinergic agonists 8
Chorea 108
Choroid plexus 53
Chronic disability, cause of 65
Churg-Strauss syndrome 51
Cingulate sulcus
  posterior half of 60f
  sign 60f
Clonazepam 77
Clonidine 8
Closed-fist sign 14
Coccidioidal meningitis 47
Coccidioides immitis 46, 47
Coccidioidomycosis 46
Cognitive impairment 65, 107, 111
Cognitive training 67
Collagen disease 13
Comorbid psychiatric illness 28
Compound muscle action potential 14, 16

Computed tomography 59
  scan 41
Condom catheters 5, 7
Conduction velocity 15
Confusion arousals 73, 77
Congenital thenar hypoplasia 13
Consolidation therapy 45
Cortical micturition center 1
Cortical venous thrombosis 108
Cotrimoxazole 41
Cranial nerve
  involvement 38
  palsy 34, 49
Creatine kinase 109
Cryptococcal disease 44
Cryptococcosis 44
Cryptococcus neoformans 44
Cunninghamella 45
Cutting food and handling utensils 102
Cyclophosphamide 50, 51
Cyclosporin A 50
Cystometrogram 4
Cystoscopy 4

D

Daily living, activities of 68
Dapsone 50
Darifenacin 7
Deep brain stimulation 30, 97
  chronic 97
Dementia 5, 57, 94, 101, 111
Dental care 96
Denture retention 96
Depression 95, 101
Detrusor
  areflexia 3
  external sphincter dyssynergia 3
  hyper-reflexia 3
  hypoactivity 6
  sphincter dyssynergia 2
Diabetes mellitus 3, 13
Diazepam 8
Dibenzyline 8
Diffusion tensor imaging 86
Digiti minimi, abductor 19
Disc
  degeneration 81
  herniation
    multiple 79f

posterolateral 81f, 82
material, superior migration of 83f
migration 79f
prolapse 81
with inferior migration, extruded l3-l4 81f
Discitis 80
Distal median motor latency 14
Domain-specific training 66
Dopamine 119
  agonists 77
Doxepin 77
Doxycycline 33, 34, 39
Dressing 102
Dysautonomic symptoms 73
Dyschondroplasia 13
Dyskinesia 75, 104
  drug-induced 98
  painful 105
  reappear 76
Dystonia
  painful 75
  presence of early morning 105

E

Echinococcosis 42
Echinococcus granulosus 42
Electroencephalography 23, 27f, 70, 108
Electromyogram 26
Electromyography 4, 15, 19, 19t, 21t, 27f
Electro-oculogram 27
Electrophysiological tests 14
Embolic strokes 126
Encephalitis 33, 34
Endoscopic third ventriculostomy 62
Endothelial nitric oxide synthase 123
Enterocystoplasty 9
Enzyme-linked immunosorbent assay 33
Eosinophilic granulomatosis 51
Epididymitis 7
Epididymorchitis 7
Epidural abscess 80
Epilepsy 22, 26, 28, 31
  syndromes 23
    genetic generalized 23

Epileptic encephalopathy 23
Epileptic seizures 27
Errorless learning 67
Eszopiclone 77
Evans' index 60
Excessive daytime sleepiness 26, 28, 73
Exploration training 69
Eye signs 113t

F

Facial expression 103
Fajersztajn's crossed sciatic sign 85
Fatigue 33, 71
Fibroblasts transplantation 10
Fibrous histiocytoma, benign 54
Fixed differential pressure valves 62, 63
Flexor carpi
 radialis 12, 19, 21
 ulnaris 12
Flexor digitorum
 profundus 12
 superficialis 12
Flexor pollicis longus 12
Flick sign 14
Flow-regulated valve 62, 63
Fluconazole 47
Flucytosine 41
Focal epilepsy syndromes 23
Frisch bacillus 38
Fungal infections 44

G

Gait 98, 104
 apraxia 58
 disturbance 57-59, 94, 100
Gamma-aminobutyric acid 8
Ganglion 13
Gastrointestinal problems 96
Globus pallidus 98
Glutamate 49
Glutamine 49
Glutathione peroxidase 124
Goiter 107
Gout 13
Granulomas 32
Granulomatosis 51
Granulomatous
 amebic encephalitis 41
 disease, idiopathic non-caseating 52
Gravity-assisted valve 62, 63
Great auricular nerve 38

H

Hakim's triad 57
Hallucinations 73, 95
Hashimotos encephalopathy 112
Headache 33, 34
Hematuria 7
Hemorrhagic stroke 127
Hepatic cholesterol synthesis 123
Herpes zoster 3, 13
High intensity 126
 statin therapy 126
Hip joint 85
Hodgkin's disease 13
Human immunodeficiency virus 36
Hydatid cyst, treatment of 42
Hydrocephalus, idiopathic normal pressure 57-59
Hygiene 102
Hyperadrenergic state 108
Hyperinsulinemia 108
Hypersensitivity 32
Hypersomnia 75
Hyperthyroidism 107
 management of 109
 neurological manifestations of 107
Hypnogram 29
Hypoglycemia 110
Hypokinesia 104
Hyponatremia 110
Hypotension 110
Hypothalamic-pituitary axis 53
Hypothenar muscles
 wasting of 13
 weakness of 13
Hypothyroid myopathy 111
Hypothyroidism 107, 110, 111
 fetal 110
 management of 111
 neonatal 110
 neurological manifestations of 110
Hypoventilation 110

I

Inching technique 15
Infectious diseases 32
Inflammatory demyelinating polyneuropathy
 acute 113
 chronic 113
Insane, general paresis of 35
Insomnia 75
 treatment of 76
Instability pain 82
Intensity
 low 126
 moderate 126
Interlaminar epidural steroid 89
Intermittent catheterization 9
Intervertebral disc 81f
Intoxication, drug 101
Intracranial intra-axial lesions 54
Intracranial pressure 61, 62
Intramedullary tumor 82f
Intraparenchymal lesions 54
Intravenous methylprednisolone 51
Isavuconazole 46, 49
Ischemic stroke 119, 125
Isoprenoid 123
 synthesis, inhibition of 123
Itraconazole 41, 45

J

Juvenile myoclonic epilepsy 23

K

Kidney ureters bladder 5
Klebsiella rhinoscleromatis 38
Kocher-Debre-Semelaigne syndrome 111
Kyphoscoliosis 87f

L

Landau-Kleffner syndrome 23
Langerhans cell histiocytosis 53, 54
 diagnosis of 54
Lasegue's sign test 85
Leflunomide 52
Leprosy 37
 multibacillary 38

Leucocyte oxidase defect 32
Leukemia 13
Levodopa 74, 97, 111
  induced dyskinesias 76
Levofloxacin 39
Levothyroxine, doses of 111
Lighthouse strategy 66
Limbic encephalitis 49
Liothyronine 110
Lipid-lowering drug 123
Lipoprotein
  low-density 123
  non-high-density 127
Liposomal amphotericin 48
Lobe epilepsy
  and parasomnia scale, frontal 25
  nocturnal
    frontal 23
    temporal 23
Low back ache 79
  chronic 88
  clinical examination 84
  electrophysiological studies 88
  epidemiology 79
  evaluation of 79, 80
  interventional therapy 89
  magnetic resonance imaging 86
  management of 79, 86, 88
  myelography 87
  neurological examination 85
  pharmacological management 88
  psychological screening 86
  radiation therapy 89
Low back pain 79, 80fc
  assessment of 87
Lumbar canal stenosis 82
  severe 79f
Lumbar lordosis, exaggeration of 79f
Lumbo-peritoneal shunt 62
Lyme disease 33

M

Magnetic resonance imaging 16, 25, 33, 34, 36, 37, 40, 41f, 42, 45, 51, 52, 59, 70
  flair 42f

functional 70
Matrix metalloproteinases 124
McAdam's diagnostic criteria 49
Melkerson-Rosenthal syndrome 38
Memory
  functional 67
  notebook 67
  training strategies 68fc
Meningitis 34
  acute 35
  basal 34
  chronic 34
Meningoencephalitis 34
Meningovascular syphilis 35, 36
Metabolic disorders 84
Metacognitive strategy training 67
Methimazole 109
Methotrexate 50, 51
Micafungin 49
Mickulicz cells 39
Micturition, supraspinal regulation of 1
Minocycline 38
Mobility 120
Mononeuritis multiplex 13
Mononuclear predominant inflammatory cells 32
Mood disorders 71
Motor abnormalities 94
Motor disability, interventions and 117
Motor dysfunction, contribution of 75
Motor examination 103
Motor fibers 3
Motor fluctuations 94
Motor neuron disease 13
Motor problems 94
Motor recovery from stroke, pharmacological medications in 118
Movement disorders 108, 111
Mucormycosis 45, 46f
Multimodal neuroenhancement, effect of 70
Myasthenia gravis 112
Mycobacterium leprae 37
Myelitis 34, 39

Myeloma, multiple 13
Myelomeningocele 3
Myelopathy 13, 34, 40
Myopathy 109
Myxedema coma 110

N

Nasal chondritis 50
Neck pain 13
Needle electromyography 15
Neonatal hypothyroidism 110
Neoplastic granulomas 53
Nerve
  compression of 12
  conduction study 18, 18f, 19, 20t
  median 14
  paralysis, quiet 37
Neurobehavioral impairments 66
Neuro-Behçet's disease 50
Neurobrucellosis 34
Neurocognitive dysfunction, treating 71
Neurodegenerative disease 54, 91
Neurodevelopmental therapy 116
Neuroenhancement tools 66, 70
Neurofeedback 70
Neurofibromatosis 13
Neurogenic bladder 1, 4t, 5, 7, 8, 8t, 9
  dysfunction 3, 5fc
  Lapides classification of 3, 3t
  management of 1
Neurogenic detrusor overactivity 3, 7
Neurogenic intrinsic sphincter deficiency 3
Neurogenic lower urinary tract dysfunction 1
Neurologic disorders 3b, 10
Neurological deficit 85fc
Neurological disease
  signs of 34
  symptoms of 34
Neuromodulation 9
Neuromuscular electrical stimulation 118
Neuropathy, silent 37

Neurorehabilitation, neuroenhancement methods of 70b
Neurorehabilitative methods 71
Neuroretinits 39
Neurosarcoidosis 52
Neurosyphilis 35
　asymptomatic 35
Nicotinamide adenine dinucleotide phosphate 123
Nightmares 73
Nitric oxide synthesis, modulation of 124
Nocturia 74
Nocturnal paresthesias 13
Nocturnal-akinesia 77
Nodular enhancing lesions, multiple 40f
Nonergot dopamine agonist 75
Noninvasive brain stimulation techniques 118
Nonminor strokes 126
Nonmotor problems 94
Nonpharmacologic therapy 98
Nonpharmacological treatment 88
Nonrapid eye movement 22, 73
Nontuberculous granulomas 54
Nuclear scans 88
Nutritional disturbances 97

O

Obstructive sleep apnea 26, 29
Occipital paroxysm 23
Occupational therapy 100
Ocular inflammation 50
Oflaxacin 38
Olfactory ensheathing cells 10
Optic atrophy 35
Orthostatic hypertension 95
Osteomyelitis 80
Osteophyte formation 83f
Oxybutynin 7, 8, 77

P

Pacemaker 87
Pachymeningitis 49
Pad test 4
Pain 13, 18
　etiology, evaluation of 80
　localized acute 83
　localized spinal 80
Panayiotopoulos syndrome 23
Panic attacks 73
Paracentral lobule 1
Parasitic infections 39
Parasomnia 75
Paraspinal region 84
Paresthesias 13, 33
Parkin-gene 92
Parkinson's disease 59, 73, 75, 91, 98
　adaptation of 98
　advanced 94, 96
　assessment scales in 101
　diagnostic criteria for 92
　disability in 100
　environmental modifications 98
　epidemiology 92
　etiological factors 92
　management of 91
　pharmacological management 94
　polysomnography in 76
　psychotherapy and counseling 100
　sleep
　　disorders in 73
　　disturbance in 75
　surgical management of 97
　unified 101t
Parkinson's patients 94, 96
Paroxysmal attacks 23, 26
Paucibacillary leprosy 38
Pelvic
　floor muscle 6
　plexus lesions 1
　trauma 3
Penile clamp 5
Pentamidine 41
Perceptual and cognitive impairment 66
Perceptual deficit, interventions for 66, 67b
Perceptual performance 66
Periodic limb movement 73
　disorder 26
　in sleep 76
Peripheral nervous system 33, 51
Peripheral neuropathy 13, 109
Pernicious anemia 3
Peroneal nerve 38
　superficial 38
Persistent axial stiffness, severe 82
Phalen's maneuver 13, 18, 20
Phalen's test 13, 14
Pharmacologic treatment 74
Pituitary bright spot, posterior 53f
Plantar fasciitis 13
Plaque, stabilization of 124
Plasmapheresis 52
Pollicis brevis, abductor 19, 21
Polyangiitis 51
Polychondritis, relapsing 49
Polycythaemia 13
Polyenes 49
Polyneuropathy 16, 111
　coexistent 16
Polysomnography 26, 29
Pontine micturition centre 1
Posaconazole 49
Positive airway pressure, continuous 30, 77
Post-Lyme disease syndrome 33
Poststroke
　aphasia 70
　depression 119
Postural tremor of hands, action of 103
Posture 104
　and alignment changes 85
Postvoid residual bladder volume 4
Pramipexole 75
Praziquantel 40, 41
Pressure hydrocephalus
　classification of normal 58fc
　normal 57, 58, 60f
　secondary normal 58
Pressure provocation test 14
Pretibial myxedema 107
Prolapsed disc material 81f
Pronator teres 19, 21
Propamidine isethionate 41
Propylthiouracil 109
Prosopagnosia 69
Prostatitis 7
Proximal median
　lesion 15
　neuropathy 13

Psychogenic nonepileptic attack disorder 26, 27
Psychosis 95
  affects 74
Pudendal nerve 1
Pulse 105t
Pure word deafness 70
Purulent lesions, chronic 48
Pyogenic granuloma 54
Pyrimethamine 43

Q

Quality of life 22

R

Radial nerves, superficial 38
Radial neuropathy 13
Radiculopathy 40
Radio iodine ablation 110
Ramelteon 77
Randomized clinical trials 8
Rapid eye movement 22, 73
  parasomnia 26
  sleep, normal 27f
Raynaud's phenomenon 13
Reactive oxygen species 124
Reflex 3
Rehabilitation 98
Renal failure 13
Renal function studies 4
Respiratory
  muscle dysfunction 74
  tract chondritis 50
Restless legs syndrome 29, 73, 76, 95
Retropulsion of fragments, L1 fracture with 84f
Rheumatoid arthritis 20
Rhinoscleroma 38
Rhizomucor 45
Rifampicin 34, 39
Rifampin 41
Rigidity, role of 75
Ring enhancing lesions, multiple 43f
Rituximab 52
Rolandic epilepsy 23
  benign 24f

S

Sacral nerve rerouting 10
Sacral spinal cord lesions 1, 2
Sacroiliac joint tenderness 85
Sarcoidosis 13, 52
Schistosoma
  haemotobium 39
  japonicum 39, 40
  mansoni 39
Schistosomiasis 39
Schwann cells 10
Sclerosis, multiple 13, 33
Seborrheic dermatitis 97
  cause of 97
Seizures 3, 34, 49, 108
Sensory
  deficit, interventions for 66
  disturbance 13
  fibers 3
  nerve 14
    action potential 16, 17
  tests, computerized quantitative 38
Sensory-evoked potentials 88
Serotonin reuptake inhibitors 116, 119
Shunt systems, types of 62
Sialorrhea 96
Sicard's sign 85
Single-photon emission computed tomography 36
Sleep 22
  apnea 74
  behavioral disorder 73
  disorders 22, 30, 73, 95
    primary 28
    treatment of 29
  disturbance 73
    symptoms of 75
  electroencephalography 30
  fragmentation 95
  latency test, multiple 29
  maintenance insomnia 75
  problems 77
  regulating structures, primary involvement of 73
  related breathing disorders 77
  terrors 23
Sleepwalking 23

Slow-wave sleep 26
Snoring 73
Soap bubble appearance 41
Solifenacin 7
Speech 98
  and language 70
    rehabilitation 71b
  therapist 96
  therapy 100
Sphincterotomy 9
Spinal cord 3, 33
  injury 3, 5
  lesions 10
    suprasacral 1, 2
  regeneration 10
  tumors 82
Spinal fibers 3
Spinal tap, routine 61
Spine
  imaging of 86
  problems, degenerative 82
Splinting 17f
Spondylolisthesis 79f, 83f
Spondylolysis 82
Spondylotic, extensive 83f
Square wrist 14
Static cystogram 4
Steroid 50, 110
  responsive encephalopathy 112
Stopping maintenance therapy 45
Straight leg raising test 85
Strategy training 68
Streptomycin 34
Stroke 3, 49, 65, 120
  and motor recovery 116
  cerebral recovery after 65
  left hemispheric 70
  management of 125
    part of 123
  nonmotor rehabilitation in 65
  patients
    fitness in 120
    rehabilitation in 116
  prevention 125
  recovery phase after 116
  severity 120
Stroke-related disability 71

Subdural hygroma 63
Sulfadiazine 43
Sulfamethoxazole 34, 43
Superoxide dismutase 124
Supraclavicular nerve 38
Suprapontine lesions 1
Suprapubic catheters 5
Suprapubic cystostomy 7
Supratentorial atrophy 54
Sural nerves 38
Swallowing problems 96
Sylvian fissure 60
Symptomatic orthostasis 105
Syphilis, advanced 3
Syphilitic meningitis, acute 35
Syringomyelia 13

T

Tabes dorsalis 35
Tactile agnosia 70
Temporal lobe epilepsy, bitemporal 23f
Tenderness and muscle spasm 84
Terazosin 8
Terminal latency index 15
Tetrahydrobiopterin 124
Thalidomide 51
Thenar eminence
  wasting of 13
  weakness of 13
Therapeutic traditional physical approach 116
Thionamides, class of 109
Thoracic outlet syndrome 13
Thought disorder 101
Thyroid
  associated eye sign 113
  associated orbitopathy sign 113, 113t
  bruit 107
  disease 107
    neurological manifestations of 113
  disorders, neurological manifestations of 107
  dysfunction 107
  hormone 107
    imbalance, neurological manifestations to 107
    replacement 111
  ophthalmopathy, management of 110
  stimulating hormone 111
Thyrotoxicosis 107
Thyrotropin-releasing hormone 111
Tibial nerves, posterior 38
Tinel's sign 13, 14
  over median nerve 13
Tingling sensations 18
Tizanidine 8
Tolterodine 7
  tartrate 8
Tonic clonic seizure 25f
  generalized 23
Topographic disorientation 69
Transcranial direct current stimulation 70, 118
Transcutaneous electrical nerve stimulation 6
Transient ischemic attacks 126
Transurethral catheters 5
Transverse myelitis 3, 5, 33
Trauma 83
Trazodone 77
Treating stroke patients 116
Tremor 98, 102
  role of 75
Treponema pallidum 35
Triceps reflexes 13
Tricyclic antidepressant 7
  drugs 8
Triggered reflex voiding 6
Trimethoprim 34
Trospium 77
  chloride 7, 8
Tuberculosis 13
Tunnel signs 41
Tunnel syndrome 13

U

Ulnar abnormalities 16
Ulnar interossei distal motor latency 15
Ulnar nerve 38
  dorsal cutaneous nerve of 38
Ulnar neuropathy 13
Ultrasonography 15
Umbilical hernia 110
Upper motor neurons 8
Urethral false passages 7
Urethral trauma 7
Urethritis 7
Urinary
  incontinence 57, 58
  tract
    infection 7, 9
    symptoms, lower 4

V

Vacuum phenomenon 83f
  compression fracture with 84f
Vagal nerve stimulation 30
  role of 30
Vanilloids 8
Vasculitides 113
Vasculitis 32, 34
Vasculopathy 113
Ventriculoatrial shunt 62
Ventriculoperitoneal shunt 62
Vesicoureteral reflux 9
Visual
  agnosia 69
  neglect 66
  restitution training 67
Visuospatial deficit, interventions for 66, 67b
Vivid dreams 73
Voriconazole 41

W

Wegner's granulomatosis 51
Wernicke's area 70
Worm-Eaten sign 41

Z

Zolpidem 77